Older People with Visual Impairment
Clinical Management and Care

Susan Watkinson

Older People with Visual Impairment Clinical Management and Care

Susan Watkinson

ISBN: 9781905539-45-1

First published 2014

British Library Cataloguing in Publication Data

A catalogue record for this book is available from the British Library

Notice

Clinical practice and medical knowledge constantly evolve. Standard safety precautions must be followed, but, as knowledge is broadened by research, changes in practice, treatment and drug therapy may become necessary or appropriate. Readers must check the most current product information provided by the manufacturer of each drug to be administered and verify the dosages and correct administration, as well as contraindications. It is the responsibility of the practitioner, utilising the experience and knowledge of the patient, to determine dosages and the best treatment for each individual patient. Any brands mentioned in this book are as examples only and are not endorsed by the publisher. Neither the publisher nor the authors assume any liability for any injury and/or damage to persons or property arising from this publication.

Disclaimer

M&K Publishing cannot accept responsibility for the contents of any linked website or online resource. The existence of a link does not imply any endorsement or recommendation of the organisation or the information or views which may be expressed in any linked website or online resource. We cannot guarantee that these links will operate consistently and we have no control over the availability of linked pages.

To contact M&K Publishing write to:

M&K Update Ltd · The Old Bakery · St. John's Street

Keswick · Cumbria CA12 5AS

Tel: 01768 773030 · Fax: 01768 781099

publishing@mkupdate.co.uk

www.mkupdate.co.uk

Designed and typeset by Mary Blood

Printed in Scotland by Bell & Bain, Glasgow

Other books from M&K include

Clinical Examination Skills for Healthcare Professionals
ISBN: 9781905539710

Routine Blood Results Explained 3/e
ISBN: 9781905539888

Understanding Chronic Kidney Disease: A guide for the non-specialist
ISBN: 9781905539741

Contents

List of figures

List of contributors

Susan Watkinson, BA, RN, OND (Hons), PGCEA, MSc (University of Surrey), PhD (University of Surrey), is an Associate Lecturer at the College of Nursing, Midwifery and Healthcare, University of West London, Brentford, London. She qualified as an ophthalmic nurse at Moorfields Eye Hospital, London where she later held Sister and Clinical Teaching posts. Ophthalmic nursing remains her specialist clinical interest and she continues to publish extensively within this field. She gained an MSc in Educational Studies and a PhD in Education from the University of Surrey. She has considerable experience of teaching ophthalmic nursing, research, and ethics and philosophy within pre- and post-registration nurse education, and research methods and applied research philosophies for post-graduate Master's Degree courses.

Mahesh Seewoodhary, BSc (Hons) Biological Sciences, RGN, OND (Hons), FETC 730, Intensive Care Certificate JBCNS, RCNT, RNT, Cert. Ed., is a Senior Lecturer in Adult Nursing at the College of Nursing, Midwifery and Healthcare, University of West London, Brentford, London. His clinical interests and expertise are in ophthalmic nursing, particularly in Accident and Emergency eye care and primary care, applied physiology and mentorship. He has published extensively in the field of ophthalmic nursing and has acted as nursing adviser to nursing journals.

Cecilia Awelewa, BSc (Hons) Professional Practice with Ophthalmic Nursing, RGN, ENB346, is Sister on the Day Surgery Prince Charles Eye Unit, King Edward VII Hospital, Windsor. She started her career as a Staff Nurse on the Prince Charles Eye Unit in 1992 and gained a BSC (Hons) in Professional Practice with Ophthalmic Nursing from Thames Valley University. Ophthalmic nursing is her specialist clinical interest. She was pivotal in the planning and implementation of nurse-led post-operative discharge in the Eye Unit. She has considerable experience in the placement and mentoring of pre- and post-registration nursing students. She currently mentors student nurses for the Degree in Nursing Programme, Adult Branch. She has been actively involved in numerous audits and publications, and is also an Associate Lecturer at the University of West London, teaching students who are undertaking Continuing Personal and Professional Development in Ophthalmic Nursing.

Foreword

This book will assist ophthalmic nurse practitioners and relevant healthcare professionals in several ways. It will enable them to develop their knowledge and enhance their expertise in the timely assessment of ophthalmic conditions of elderly patients. It will also help them in the appropriate management of individuals who are visually impaired due to age-related ocular diseases. Finally, it will improve their ability to deal with organisational challenges involving visually impaired elderly patients, and consider their future treatment and management.

Sue Watkinson has incorporated her broad professional and academic knowledge relating to ophthalmic nursing and advanced nursing professional practice issues in order to analyse the multiplicity of nursing roles involved in caring for elderly individuals with visual impairment due to age-related ocular diseases. All the key age-related ocular diseases, including cataract, age-related macular degeneration, chronic open-angle glaucoma, diabetic retinopathy and dementia, are presented.

The book begins by discussing the pathogenesis, clinical features, aetiology, risk factors, classification and diagnosis of age-related ocular diseases. The author and contributors go on to draw links between age-related ocular diseases and changes related to demographics, health policy and the economy in order to highlight the psychosocial impact of these changes on the quality of life for elderly individuals with ocular disease.

As in her previous work, Sue Watkinson plunges deeply into the field of ophthalmic care issues. In particular, she progressively sketches and stretches the role of specialist ophthalmic nurses in informing and educating patients, the management of ophthalmic treatment procedures, the promotion of safe environments and the maintenance of quality of life for elderly individuals suffering from age-related ophthalmic conditions.

Finally, the book makes a very important contribution by outlining advanced and specialist roles for ophthalmic nurses practising in both primary and community-based settings, thus enhancing the quality of care, service and management of age-related ocular diseases.

Dr Stefanos Mantzoukas
(RGN, BSc Nurs., BSc Health Stud., PgCert.T&L, PgDip SRM, MSc, PhD, FEANS)
Assistant Professor in Nursing, Epirus Institute of Technology, Greece
Honorary Lecturer in the MPH programme, University of Liverpool, UK
Online Tutor in Nursing, University of Derby, UK

Acknowledgements

The author would like to thank all those involved in the production process, especially my commissioning editor, Mike Roberts. I would also like to acknowledge the valuable contributions from Ramesh Seewoodhary and Cecilia Awelewa in Chapters 2 and 6.

Finally, I wish to thank both my academic and clinical colleagues for their continued moral support during the writing of this book. Special thanks to Chris Robinson at the University of West London for his initial valuable help with image preparation.

Preface

Older People with Visual Impairment presents some current perspectives on managing the care of older people with visual impairment due to age-related ocular disease. The major age-related ocular diseases in the United Kingdom include cataract, age-related macular degeneration, chronic open-angle glaucoma and diabetic retinopathy. This book also presents an overview of some of the significant issues affecting this area of practice including demographic change, health policy, epidemiology of sight loss, the cost of sight loss for the UK economy and the psychosocial impact of losing sight. All these issues make caring for older people with visual impairment more challenging.

The book will be of benefit to all ophthalmic and general nurses working in hospital wards, accident and emergency departments, eye centres, eye clinics, nursing homes, residential care homes, in older people's own homes in the community, primary care practice nurses, district nurses, community mental health nurses, social workers, occupational therapists, healthcare assistants, support workers and student nurses.

It is also important to stress that, as technology advances, specialist nurses with a high level of competence and technical skill are pivotal to achieving successful outcomes in the safe and effective delivery of care to older people with visual impairment, within a culture of compassion, commitment and strong leadership.

The author of this book hopes to draw the reader's attention to the importance of meeting the individual needs of older people as the cornerstone of a patient-centred approach to care. Providing the appropriate care for this vulnerable group of people in our society will help reduce the economic and psychological burden of sight loss and re-establish a good quality of life for the older person with visual impairment.

Introduction
Ageing and the needs of older people
Susan Watkinson

This short introduction provides a background to the main text by looking at some definitions of ageing and 'the older person'. It describes the general and obvious characteristics of ageing, followed by the specific clinical features of advancing age with reference to the main systems of the body. It emphasises the importance of the role of the nurse and other relevant health and social care professionals in adopting a holistic approach to caring for older people with visual impairment by identifying both their physical and psychological needs in diverse healthcare settings.

Defining ageing
Ageing is a gradual and continuous process and can be described in various ways. It may be seen as a distinct and progressive decline in function, which makes a person more vulnerable to disease, or a process leading to functional impairment of tissues and organs (Tortora and Derrickson, 2013). It may also be seen as a series of changes leading to the loss of function of organs and cells, eventually resulting in death. Life expectancy in the developed world is now 80 years for females, and 75 years for males (Tortora and Derrickson, 2013).

Defining the 'older person'
Most developed-world countries accept the chronological age of 65 years as a definition of 'elderly' or 'older person'. Whilst it might be argued that this is somewhat arbitrary, it is often associated with the age at which a person begins to receive pension benefits (World Health Organisation (WHO) 2013). Currently, there is no United Nations standard numerical criterion, but it is agreed that the cut-off point is 60 years and above to refer to the older population. The American Psychological Association (2014) affirms that older adults are defined as 65 years of age and older, and that the 'oldest old' group (that is, those aged 85 years and older) is increasing faster than any other age group. For the purposes of this text, an older person will be taken to mean a person aged 65 years and above.

The characteristics of ageing
The obvious characteristics of ageing are: greying and loss of hair, loss of teeth, wrinkling

1

of skin, decreased muscle mass, and increased fat deposits (Tortora & Derrickson 2013). Physiologically, there is a gradual deterioration in function and capacity to respond to environmental stress. Basic kidney function and digestive metabolic rates decrease and there is a diminished ability to respond effectively to changes in temperature, diet and oxygen supply to maintain a constant internal environment. Such manifestations of ageing are related to an overall decrease in the number of body cells and to the less effective functioning of remaining cells. Thousands of brain cells are lost daily (Tortora & Derrickson 2013).

The ageing process within the body

The main systems of the body will now be considered (adapted from Tortora & Derrickson 2013).

Cardiovascular system

Changes due to ageing include loss of extensibility of the aorta, reduction in cardiac cell size, progressive loss of cardiac muscular strength, reduced cardiac output, and an increase in blood pressure. Changes in the blood vessels, such as hardening of arteries and cholesterol deposits in arteries serving brain tissue, reduce nourishment to the brain, resulting in its malfunction or death of brain tissues.

Respiratory system

With advancing age, the airways and tissues of the respiratory tract become less elastic and more rigid, resulting in a decrease in pulmonary lung capacity. The vital capacity (the amount of air moved by maximal inspiration, followed by maximal expiration) can be reduced by as much as 35% by the age of 70. There is also a decrease in blood levels of oxygen, reduced activity of alveolar macrophages, and diminished ciliary action of the epithelium lining the respiratory tract. The consequence of such age-related changes means that older people are more susceptible to pneumonia, bronchitis, emphysema and other pulmonary diseases.

Genito-urinary tract

By the age of 80, between 10% and 30% of the glomeruli in the kidneys no longer work. Around 25% of the kidney mass is lost, due to shrivelling of the outer part of the kidney. Generally, the kidneys are still able to regulate the fluid levels in the body, and reduced function will only be apparent at times of physical stress.

Urinary incontinence and urinary tract infections are two major problems associated with ageing. Changes and diseases in the kidney include acute and chronic kidney inflammations and renal calculi. The prostate gland is often implicated in various disorders of the urinary tract, and cancer of the prostate gland is the most frequent malignancy in males. Benign enlargement of the prostate gland occurs in 25–50% of men over 65. This leads to incomplete emptying of the bladder and a weak stream of urine or signs of irritation with frequency of urination.

Liver

During the ageing process, there will be a 25% reduction in liver mass, although function remains within normal limits. Protein production will be slightly reduced and there will be an impaired metabolism of some drugs through the liver.

Immune system

With age, the immune system changes and becomes more dysfunctional. The thymus gland, situated behind the sternum, has an important role to play in immunity. Normally, its function is to transform lymphocytes (white blood cells developed in the bone marrow) into T-cells, which destroy invading microbes directly or indirectly by producing various substances and generally help to combat infection.

With age, this gland shrinks, resulting in a greatly reduced immune function. Infectious disease (such as bronchopneumonia and influenza) is ten times more likely to be the cause of death in the elderly, and older people are more likely to experience a reactivation of certain diseases such as herpes zoster (shingles) and tuberculosis. There is also an increased occurrence of autoimmune diseases and cancers.

Neurosensory system

In this system there is a loss of neurons in the brain and spinal cord and loss of neuronal dendrites, which reduces the amount of synaptic transmission. The senses of smell, taste, sight, touch and hearing are all diminished over time. Depression can also be the result of impaired synaptic activity. Research indicates that as many as 25% of nursing home residents are clinically depressed. Depression is one of the most common causes of weight loss.

Eyes

With specific reference to the eyes, it is essential for certain changes to be observed and understood in the older person. The lens hardens, causing presbyopia (difficulty in focusing on near objects), and from around the age of 40 onwards people find that they need to wear reading glasses to help them focus more clearly. The retina becomes less sensitive to light, which makes it harder for older people to read in low or dim light and to distinguish low-contrast objects from each other. The pupils also react more slowly. This means that elderly people have difficulty adjusting to changes in light levels.

For the older person, this could result in difficulty with night driving. Peripheral and colour vision may become less sensitive with age. A change in peripheral vision is due to a smaller pupil, a more opaque lens and a less sensitive retina, whilst a change in colour perception will be the result of a yellowing of the lens, which occurs with old age.

Ears

A decline in hearing is a very common age-related change. Impaired hearing exists in a third of older people aged 65 and over, and in 80% of 80-year-olds. This is a condition known as presbyacusis.

Muscle

With ageing there is a decrease in muscular strength and power, and lean body mass (up to 30 to 40%). There is also an increase in fat body mass. This process is known as sarcopenia and results in decreased functional capacity.

Skin

The skin becomes more fragile and susceptible to damage. Wound healing takes longer. The fat layer decreases, but fat accumulates in particular areas (such as the stomach and under the chin). Pigment cells are fewer but clump together, giving the appearance of paler skin with age spots. The skin gets drier and more susceptible to flakiness; the sense of pain is lessened and temperature regulation is less efficient. Hair and nail growth slow down, hair thins, nails thicken and become yellower. The skin is less able to withstand infections and malignant change as the immune function declines. Skin becomes dry and itchy and bruises easily.

Bones

With advancing age, osteoporosis can set in. This is a reduction of bone mass with a deterioration of bone tissue, causing increased fragility of the bones and a susceptibility to fracture. Women are especially affected after the menopause; the condition affects men more slowly. With increasing age, blood calcium comes from bone more than diet. Calcium supplements combined with Vitamin D can be very helpful in this age group and have been found to reduce the incidence of falls in patients living in residential care homes.

The needs of older people

The needs of older people are probably best identified by asking the older people themselves. Some interesting results have emerged from the work of Kydd et al. (2009), in which older people identified seven main attributes as being desirable in a healthcare professional. These are, in order of importance:

● A caring, understanding and kind person
● A professional attitude to older people

- A patient person who will listen
- A respectful person
- A skilful, knowledgeable practitioner
- Continuity of care
- A cheerful person.

In summary, caring, understanding and kindness took priority over skill. Older people wanted a person whose time was dictated by a patient's needs, not by a schedule. A healthcare professional with a positive attitude to working with older people was also viewed as important, and someone who could understand that age or infirmity did not necessarily mean an inability to participate in informed decisions concerning their own healthcare.

Generally, a 70-year-old cannot do what a 30-year-old can, even when they are essentially fit. However, an older person is still an individual, and individuality and dignity are just as important to older people as they are to the young.

Patience and taking time to listen were seen as very important attributes. Older people wanted the healthcare professional to listen to their expectations and requirements and discuss what is and is not possible. Older people preferred a healthcare professional to ask how they would like to be addressed, rather than automatically referring to them by their first names. This was felt to be disrespectful by some older people. Also, as part of showing respect, there needs to be a realisation that age, frail health or limited mobility may still be accompanied by an active mind and one which likes to engage in normal conversation.

Older people wanted a practitioner who made an effort to ascertain what suited their individual needs with reference to their illness, social circumstances and rehabilitation. It was important to have someone who could provide answers to their questions and advise them how to cope when they returned home from hospital or residential care. Reference was also made to receiving fragmented care, which was viewed as poor practice.

The idea of having regular visits by the same healthcare professional, as far as possible, promoted comfort and engagement and made it easier to communicate with the carer about their own family and the outside world. Finally, older people wanted to see a happy, cheerful and willing healthcare professional. A bright and happy attitude when dealing with general daily queries was felt to be a very special quality in a healthcare professional. Indeed, many found the presence of cheerful healthcare professionals very therapeutic.

The role of health and social care professionals

From this data, we can conclude that what has been viewed as older people's expectations of their healthcare professionals, with reference to the identification and fulfilment of their needs, is already embedded in the Nursing and Midwifery Council (2009) guidance for practice in the care of older people. Here, the approach to care is summarised as getting to know and value older people as individuals, finding out how they want to be cared for, and providing care that promotes respect, dignity and fairness.

From this introductory discussion, it seems clear that one of the most important aspects of caring for older people is being able to conduct a detailed assessment that identifies their needs as members of a distinct age group in order to provide individualised care. This means adopting a holistic approach and considering the older person as a complete individual, both physically and psychologically. Anything that has an impact on their health and well-being should be considered when determining how best to deliver individualised care. Clearly, it is essential for all health and social care professionals caring for older people to have sound knowledge and understanding of the physiological and psychological changes taking place due to ageing and, more importantly, to apply that knowledge to the planning and delivery of their care.

Older people from black and minority ethnic groups

It is also important for health and social care professionals to consider the specific needs of older people from black and minority ethnic (BME) groups as part of a detailed and holistic assessment of the older person. Problems commonly faced by BME groups include lack of information, lack of awareness of information or other available services, language barriers and/or culturally inappropriate services and information. BME populations are the highest users of primary care health services, yet they are less likely to gain access to appropriate health services and treatment and they report the worst health outcomes. Their usage of community health services also tends to be low.

More specifically, they will be the least likely to seek help when suffering sight problems even though they are often the most vulnerable to losing sight. For example, Asian people have a greater risk of developing cataract compared with the black and white populations. People of African-Caribbean descent are eight times more likely to develop glaucoma than the general population and it tends to occur in them 10 to 15 years earlier than in other ethnic groups. Black and Asian populations also have a greater risk of developing diabetic eye disease compared to the white population.

To conclude, this book discusses older people with visual impairment who are receiving treatment in a variety of healthcare settings, including hospitals, eye centres, eye clinics, nursing homes, residential care homes, and in their own homes within the community. However, regardless of the setting, health and social care professionals caring for older people with visual impairment will be applying the same basic principles of care, and identifying and dealing with the specific needs associated with visual impairment due to major ocular disease.

References

American Psychological Association (2014). 'Practitioners Working With Older Adults'. APA Working Group on the Older Adult Brochure: Executive Summary.
www.apa.org/pi/aging/resources/guides/practitioners-should-know.aspx (Last accessed: 10 April 2014).

Kydd, A., Duffy, T. & Duffy, R. (eds) (2009). *The Care and Wellbeing of Older People.* Devon: Reflect Press.

Nursing and Midwifery Council (2009). *Guidance: for the care of older people.*
www.nmc-uk.org/documents/guidance/guidance-for-the-care-of-older-people.pdf (Last accessed: 10 April 2014).

Tortora, G.J. & Derrickson, B.H. (2013). *Essentials of Anatomy and Physiology.* Ninth Edition International Student Version. Singapore: John Wiley & Sons Singapore Pte. Ltd.

World Health Organisation (2013). *Definition of an older or elderly person.*
www.who.int/healthinfo/survey/ageingdefnolder/en/
(Last accessed: 17 April 2014).

Chapter 1

Older people with visual impairment: Clinical management and care – an overview

Susan Watkinson

This chapter covers

- Introduction
- Demographic change and health policy
- Older people with dementia
- Sight loss and its economic impact
- Major age-related ocular diseases in the UK
- Psychosocial impact of sight loss
- The nursing role in managing older people with visual impairment
- Creating the right culture within the NHS
- Conclusion.

Introduction

This book focuses exclusively on older people with significant age-related ocular disease within the United Kingdom. The text therefore begins by examining the main age-related ocular diseases that give rise to visual impairment in this section of the population: cataract, age-related macular degeneration, chronic open-angle glaucoma and diabetic retinopathy. Some commonly occurring external ocular conditions affecting older people, including dry eyes, ectropion, entropion and blepharitis, will be addressed in Chapter 6. The second important focus will be on the principles of care that should be embraced by all health and social care professionals when caring for older people with visual impairment in diverse settings such as hospitals, eye centres, eye clinics, nursing and residential care homes, and their own homes.

This chapter gives an overview of some significant issues affecting this area of practice, including demographic change, health policy, the epidemiology of sight loss, the cost of sight loss for the UK economy, and the psychological impact of sight loss. This will serve as a useful backdrop to facilitate the reader's understanding of the challenging nature of managing the care of older people with visual impairment due to the major age-related ocular diseases listed above.

Demographic change and health policy

Clearly, the population of the UK is ageing. The percentage of the population aged 65 and over has increased from 15% in 1985, to 17% in 2010, an increase of 1.7 million people. This trend is set to continue. By 2035, 23% of the population is projected to be aged 65 and over, compared to 18% under 16 (UK National Statistics Publication Hub 2014). The fastest population increase has been in the number of those aged 85 and over, currently referred to as the 'oldest old'.

Numbers have more than doubled since 1985 and reached 1.4 million in 2010. It is estimated that, by 2031, 27.2 million people will be over the age of 50 and the over-85 age group will constitute 3.8% of the UK population (UK National Statistics Publication Hub 2014). By 2035, the number of people aged 85 and over is projected to reach 3.6 million, accounting for 5% of the total population (UK National Statistics Publication Hub 2014).

Such projections will inevitably mean an increase in the incidence of sight problems, since visual impairment is largely an age-related phenomenon (Watkinson 2009a). Eye care must be regarded as an integral component of the healthcare of older people (Royal National Institute of Blind People 2013a). The UK Vision Strategy 2013–2018 (RNIB 2013a), a VISION 2020 UK initiative led by the RNIB, has identified three strategy outcomes to set the direction for eye health and sight loss services for the next five years (see Box 1.1).

Box 1.1: The strategy outcomes of the UK Vision Strategy 2013–2018

Strategy outcome 1:
Everyone in the UK looks after their eyes and sight.

Strategy outcome 2:
Everyone with an eye condition receives timely treatment and, if permanent sight loss occurs, early and appropriate services and support are available and accessible to all.

Strategy outcome 3:
A society in which people with sight loss can fully participate.
(RNIB 2013a)

The over-arching aims of the UK Vision Strategy include:

- Raising awareness and understanding of eye health, with a particular emphasis on people most at risk of eye disease
- Encouraging every individual to develop personal responsibility for their eye health and sight
- Raising awareness of eye health and the impact of sight loss among health and social care practitioners and ensuring early detection of sight loss and prevention where possible
- Improving the co-ordination, integration, reach and effectiveness of eye health and eye care services
- Ensuring that, when permanent sight loss occurs, emotional support, habilitation and/or rehabilitation will be provided in a timely fashion, enabling people to retain or regain their independence
- Improving attitudes, awareness and actions within education, employment and other services
- Achieving improved compliance with equality legislation.

(Adapted from RNIB 2013a)

The UK Vision Strategy is positive in content but remains a challenging framework for the transformation of eye health, eye care and sight loss services across the UK, especially in the current difficult financial climate. It is to be hoped that future implementation of services at national and local level will help to drive forward the priorities of the Vision Strategy. Providing specialist care to improve eye health screening and low vision services has been a priority for the government, but it must continue its drive to deliver a comprehensive service that also keeps further cost to the taxpayer to a minimum.

Older people with dementia

It is a cause of considerable concern that the number of older people with dementia who will also become visually impaired is set to increase for the future.

Dementia currently costs the UK economy about £23 billion per year. This is twice the cost of cancer, three times the cost of heart disease and four times the cost of stroke (Luengo-Fernandez et al. 2010). Estimates of the number of people currently living with dementia in the UK range from around 684,000 to 822,000.

Among these older people it is thought that approximately 15,000 are from minority ethnic groups (DH 2009a). Although population ageing means that the number of people with dementia overall will increase, the number of black and minority ethnic (BME) older people with dementia will grow even more sharply. The frequency of dementia rises with age and the number of BME older people in their seventies and eighties is growing steadily (Lievesley 2010). Therefore, this is likely to lead to an increased need for dementia services. Currently, however, BME older people are under-represented in dementia services due to lower levels of awareness about dementia and the existence of stigma associated with it within BME communities (Moriarty et al. 2011). The incidence of visual impairment in BME older people will similarly increase. No reference has been made, however, to the need for eye care provision in the recent National Dementia Strategy for England (DH 2009a).

Diagnosis of visual impairment in older people with dementia is nevertheless important in order to ensure the maximum effectiveness of their treatment and care, since sensory deprivation profoundly increases the sense of disorientation (Jones & Trigg 2007). A more detailed discussion of the needs of older people with dementia and visual impairment, and the implications for their care and management, is provided in Chapter 9 of this book. Other associated problems of dementia, such as depression and difficulty with communicating and performing daily living activities (DH 2009a), which compound failing vision, will also be discussed in Chapter 9.

With the predicted increase in the number of older people over the next three decades, the continued funding of the cost of treating major ocular disease has to remain speculative for the future (Watkinson 2009a). The implications of continued financial constraint over the next decade may result in the UK government being unable to meet the key NHS priority for the healthcare of older people with sight impairment. Furthermore, such constraint may continue to result in a decline in the numbers of qualified practitioners, which may compromise the delivery of high standards of care for the future.

It is already apparent that the employment of healthcare assistants and support workers will offer a cheaper option for the future. Such workers will be providing basic care and services for the ever-expanding vulnerable group of older people within our society (Watkinson 2009b). Certainly, this situation raises many issues for debate, the full extent of which are beyond the scope of this text. However, some concluding thoughts on the key issues, including the need to train healthcare workers, the need for adequate supervision of such workers by qualified nurses, and the role of mentorship, will be offered in the concluding chapter of this book.

Sight loss and its economic impact

Almost two million people in the UK are living with sight loss (RNIB 2013b). One in five people aged 75 years and over are living with sight loss and it is a ratio of one in two people for those aged 90 years and over. Nearly two-thirds of people with sight loss are women, and people from black and ethnic minority communities are at greater risk of some of the leading causes of sight loss. Furthermore, adults with learning disabilities are 10 times more likely to be blind or partially sighted than the general population (RNIB 2013b). Future projections also indicate that the numbers of people with sight problems in the UK are likely to increase dramatically over the next 25 years. By 2020, those people with sight loss will have risen to over 2,250,000. By 2050, this figure will have almost doubled to nearly four million (RNIB 2013b).

Clearly, sight loss is very expensive, both for society and the individual. In 2008, for example, the cost of sight loss, excluding that in children, was at least £6.5 billion. This cost was made up of £2.14 billion in direct healthcare costs, such as eye clinics, prescriptions and operations; £4.34 billion comprised indirect costs such as unpaid carer costs and reduced employment rates (Access Economics 2009). Sight loss also has a major impact on quality of life and this was also measured using the disability adjusted life years approach (Access Economics 2009). The outcome of this research was that a monetary value of £15.5 billion was placed on the quality of life lost due to sight loss. Overall, the direct, indirect and quality of life costs of sight loss in the UK amounted to £22 billion in 2008.

With specific reference to age-related ocular disease, Minassian & Reidy (2009) used an incidence-based approach to measure the costs of sight loss. They focused on four main treatable causes of sight loss – namely age-related macular degeneration (AMD), cataract, diabetic retinopathy and glaucoma – to estimate the number of people experiencing sight loss from each disease in the base year (2010). The baseline cost of AMD in 2010 was estimated to be £1.6 billion, £0.99 billion for cataract, £0.68 billion for diabetic retinopathy and £0.54 billion for glaucoma. The cumulative total cost for these four eye diseases through to 2020 is estimated to be over £37 billion (Minassian & Reidy 2009). An overview of these four main ocular diseases will now be given.

Major age-related ocular diseases in the UK

The four major ocular diseases and causes of blindness in the UK are cataract, chronic open-angle glaucoma (COAG), AMD and diabetic retinopathy and 50% of all sight problems in patients aged over 65 years are due to untreated cataracts or refractive error (WHO 2007).

Estimates based on official population projections and epidemiological prevalence surveys predict that the number of cases of glaucoma in England and Wales will increase by a third by 2021, and then continue to rise at a similar rate by 2031 (DH 2009b). Clearly, preventing visual impairment and blindness in older people is a key aim for government health policy. Currently, 'blindness' is defined as visual acuity of less than 3/60 or a corresponding visual field loss to less than 10 degrees in the better eye with the best possible correction. 'Visual impairment' includes both low vision and blindness (WHO 2007).

Cataract

Cataract is a common world-wide cause of visual impairment, and cataract surgery continues to be the elective surgical procedure most commonly performed in the UK (Royal College of Ophthalmologists 2010), where approximately 330,000 cataract operations are performed each year. In the UK, cataract surgery is performed as same-day surgery under local anaesthetic, with a six-week recovery period. It is predominantly performed on older patients – with over 90% being 60 years of age or older, and just under 60% being 75 years or older.

With continuing advances in microsurgical techniques and intra-ocular lens technology, the quality of post-operative optical rehabilitation has also continued to improve, which has in turn influenced the indications for surgery. The demand for cataract surgery has thus continued to increase. With demographic change and the predicted increase in the number of older people, both the prevalent cases of cataract and the demand for surgery will continue to rise (RCO 2010). In fact, from 2010 to 2050, the share of partial sight and blindness arising from cataract in the UK is predicted to increase from 13.7% to 15.2%; that is, to 600,000 people (RNIB 2009b).

Undoubtedly, cataract visual impairment can have a major negative impact on the quality of older people's lives. In Chapter 2, consideration will therefore be given to some of the important issues associated with managing the care of older people with cataracts, as well as offering some key perspectives on how technology has advanced current approaches to treatment in order to restore a sighted quality of life.

Age-related macular degeneration

AMD is a major cause of ocular morbidity in high-income countries, accounting for over half of blind and partial sight certifications in the UK (Bunce et al. 2010). In 2010, a total of 608,213 people in the UK were estimated to have AMD and this is expected to increase to 755,867 by the end of the decade (Minassian et al. 2011). Numbers with sight loss from AMD are expected to rise from 223,224 in 2010 to 291,982 by 2020. Cases with sight loss due to neovascular AMD are expected to increase from 145,697 to 189,890 by the end of the decade (Minassian et al. 2011).

Such statistical predictions give some indication of the scale of health and social service provision required for older people with AMD and the cost of treatment for the future. Furthermore, Minassian et al.'s (2011) findings indicate that the beneficial effects of anti-vascular endothelial growth factor (VEGF) therapy, the current treatment of choice, would be outweighed by the strong anticipated demographic 'ageing' effect. This also reaffirms the importance of continuing efforts to develop more effective and more broadly applicable therapies for AMD. The main issues and debates surrounding AMD, and the clinical management of older people with this condition, are discussed in detail in Chapter 3.

Chronic open-angle glaucoma

COAG affects older people as a chronic condition that requires lifetime monitoring and management (Watkinson 2009b). Prevalence increases with age, and the number affected is estimated to rise to almost 10% in people over 75. The prevalence may also be higher in people of black African or black Caribbean descent or those with a family history of glaucoma. It is estimated that around 489,000 people are currently affected by COAG in England (NICE 2009). There are an estimated 11,054 cases of COAG in people aged 40 to 70 each year in the UK. The number for England is an estimated 9,263 new cases of COAG per year (NICE 2009).

After AMD, COAG is one of the principal reasons for having to register as blind; in fact, approximately 10% of UK blindness registrations are attributed to glaucoma (NICE 2009). Clearly, this will have a resource impact at local level for the future. More detailed discussion of managing older people with COAG is provided in Chapter 4.

Diabetic retinopathy

It has been estimated that diabetes may be responsible for at least 5% of healthcare expenditure in the UK, and up to 10% of hospital budgets are used for people with diabetes (NICE 2008). It is of great concern that more than half a million people with diabetes in England are at increased risk of blindness because they have not received retinal screening, an essential annual check for the presence of diabetic retinopathy (Diabetes UK 2012).

Diabetic retinopathy is the leading cause of blindness in the UK's working population and it is one complication that people with diabetes could be at risk of developing because they are missing out on a wide range of health checks and specialist services (Diabetes UK 2012). More discussion of the importance of retinal screening as part of the clinical management of older people with diabetic retinopathy is provided in Chapter 5.

Psychosocial impact of sight loss

Visual impairment affects health-related quality of life by restricting functional ability, as well as having a detrimental effect on the psychosocial status of individuals. Clearly, the psychosocial impact is substantial (see Low Vision Service Model Evaluation Project, RNIB 2009c). Evans et al.'s (2007) study reported an association between visual impairment and depression in 13,900 people aged 75 in the UK, who had been randomly selected for health screening from 49 GP practices.

More recently, in a systematic review of research into the effects of vision loss on mental health and social functioning of older adults (aged 60 and over), Nyman et al. (2010) looked at seven outcomes: depression/mental health, anxiety, quality of life, social functioning, loneliness, social support and interventions. There were seven key findings, the most significant of which was that older people with vision loss are more at risk of reporting symptoms of depression and lower mental health, and being diagnosed with clinical depression, than their sighted peers. Furthermore, visual functioning (rather than visual status) has a stronger link with depressive symptoms. Overall, their findings reflected complex relationships among the outcomes. Importantly, they concluded that interventions directly addressing psychosocial needs are more effective than those addressing them indirectly through the use of scales to assess the degree of depression and the level of psychosocial need (Nyman et al. 2010).

In the rest of this book, the psychosocial effects of visual impairment are addressed, with reference to the presenting ocular disease under consideration. Chapter 8 in particular, focuses in more detail on the relationship between depression and visual impairment and its implications for older people, with reference to AMD, COAG and diabetic retinopathy. Here it is also argued that for the future the primary challenge for nurses is recognition of the patient's condition, which is pivotal to providing appropriate treatment. As a sobering prelude to this discussion, it is estimated that 30% of patients with AMD will experience depression within a few months of their second eye becoming affected (Preventing Depression in Age-Related Macular Degeneration (AMD) Trial 2007).

In patients with diabetes mellitus, depression has been linked to increased hyperglycaemic episodes, increased vascular complications, including diabetic retinopathy, and even increased mortality (Shahid 2012). Furthermore, patients with glaucoma and depression are less likely to use prescribed eye drops as instructed, and patients undergoing laser photocoagulation for diabetic retinopathy are more likely to associate this treatment with pain, and thus less likely to return for follow-up care (Shahid 2012).

The nursing role in managing older people with visual impairment

From the discussion so far, it is clear that visual impairment in older people presents both current and future challenges for all health and social care professionals working in hospitals, eye centres, eye clinics, nursing and residential care homes and in the community, since sight loss is largely age-related. Early diagnosis and prompt treatment are therefore instrumental in improving or preserving sight for as long as possible and providing the older person with a better sight-related quality of life.

Undoubtedly, all health and social care professionals continue to play an important role as health educators in providing older people with relevant information and help and support to gain sufficient control over the management of their visual problems. This helps to re-establish sighted quality of life and thus restore and maintain the older person's self-esteem and confidence (Seewoodhary & Watkinson, 2009).

The healthcare professional's knowledge and understanding of the major ocular diseases and the resulting visual loss, together with an appreciation of their impact on the ability to perform daily living activities, is essential for the effective planning and provision of care for older people. This can only be achieved by meeting individual needs and by providing information about available treatments, support groups and low vision services (Seewoodhary & Watkinson 2009). Indeed, the provision of high-quality patient-centred care is a key priority for the NHS (DH 2009).

Health and social care professionals are likely to encounter older people more frequently than any other age group in the future. Consequently, visual impairment in older people will present many challenges for developing the health professional's role in practice in order to meet growing demands for delivery of both primary and community-based eye health services (Watkinson 2009b). Important factors will therefore need to be considered. These include advancing their professional knowledge base related to practice, developing effective communication and counselling skills, and demonstrating knowledge and understanding of patients' ethical and legal rights in their role as patient advocates in the decision-making process.

Overall, there is a need to continue to advance practice and deliver high-quality care for older people with visual impairment. Importantly, these requirements need to be met not only by qualified practitioners but also by healthcare assistants and support workers, who will be delivering the basic care. However, this raises many issues, such as the need to train healthcare workers, their adequate supervision by qualified nurses, and mentorship. Such issues will be key challenges for the future delivery of ophthalmic care in the UK. However, whilst they are important to address, they are beyond the scope of this book. Meanwhile, creating the right culture (a strategy that is currently being pursued within the NHS) is very pertinent to all healthcare practitioners involved in managing the care of older people with visual impairment.

Creating the right culture within the NHS

Following the recommendations of the Francis Report (DH 2013), healthcare practitioners are being encouraged to revisit and reinforce the values, beliefs and behaviours that underpin their caring practice wherever it takes place (DH 2012). Such values and behaviours are seemingly embodied in the concept of the 6Cs and are heralded as the cornerstone of patient-centred care. The 6Cs include: Care, Compassion, Competence, Communication, Courage and Commitment.

Delivering this vision will be driven by commitment to six proposed areas of action (see Table 1.1) where concentrated effort will result in positive outcomes for patients. Significantly, there will be an emphasis on the areas that will have the biggest impact for the whole population and particularly for older people.

Table 1.1: Six areas of action for delivering the vision strategy

---

1. Helping people to stay independent, maximising well-being and improving health outcomes
2. Working with people to provide a positive experience of care
3. Delivering high quality care and measuring the impact of care
4. Building and strengthening leadership
5. Ensuring the right staff, with the right skills, in the right place
6. Supporting positive staff experience.

(DH 2012)

Clearly, creating the right organisational culture is pivotal to achieving high-quality care. This involves encouraging healthcare staff to challenge the status quo, work to improve quality and patient and user experience, and promote an environment in which staff can help deliver the best care for patients. This culture is crucial for embedding the concept of the 6Cs. Conceivably, this strategy presents a positive professional ideology for the future. Nevertheless, some counter-arguments may be raised concerning the potential constraints of working within this ideological framework in practice and the implications for the reality of caring for older patients with visual impairment. Arguably, providing strong and effective leadership at all levels is probably the most significant area of action required to improve organisational culture.

With specific reference to nursing older people, similar guiding principles of practice have been offered in the areas of people, process and place (NMC 2009). The first principle is that nurses must be capable of delivering safe and effective care for older people, and this is especially relevant for those older people with sight loss. The second principle is to deliver quality care that promotes dignity by nurturing and supporting the older person's self-respect and self-worth. Again, this is also relevant for nurses caring for older people with impaired vision. The third principle is that any setting that provides care for older people should be adequately resourced and should provide an appropriate and safe environment in which to practise dignified care. Furthermore, there should be strong leadership from managers capable of setting and maintaining standards of care and supporting their healthcare teams through training, development, supervision and reflection (NMC 2009).

Conclusion

In summary, this first chapter has attempted to clarify the main aims of this book by providing a structural outline and brief overview. It has also offered a brief introduction to the major age-related ocular diseases currently in the UK and signposted their further discussion in subsequent chapters with reference to current approaches to the treatment and management of older people with visual impairment.

To provide some background to the whole area of managing older people with visual impairment, this first chapter also discussed some significant issues such as demographic change, health policy, the epidemiology of sight loss, the costs of sight loss for the UK economy, and the psychosocial impact of sight loss. Such issues will inevitably influence the future delivery of care. It is hoped that this scene setting will have facilitated the reader's knowledge and understanding of the main age-related ocular diseases discussed in this text, and will also have given an appreciation of some of the complexities and challenges of managing the care of older patients with visual impairment for the remainder of the twenty-first century. In Chapter 2, a detailed overview of cataract and current perspectives on managing older people with cataracts will be presented.

References

Access Economics (2009). Future Sight Loss UK 1: *Economic Impact of Partial Sight and Blindness in the UK Adult Population.* London: Royal National Institute of Blind People.

Bunce, C., Xing, W. & Wormald, R. (2010). Causes of blind and partial sight certification in England and Wales: April 2007–March 2008. *Eye* (London). **24**, 1692–9.

Department of Health (2009a). *Living Well with Dementia: A National Dementia Strategy.* London: DH.

Department of Health (2009b). *Primary Care and Community Services: Improving Eye Health Services.* London: DH.

Department of Health (2012). *Compassion in Practice. Nursing, Midwifery and Care Staff. Our Vision and Strategy.* London: NHS Commissioning Board.

Department of Health (2013). *Independent Inquiry into Care provided by Mid Staffordshire NHS Foundation Trust: January 2005–March 2009.* The Mid Staffordshire NHS Foundation Trust Public Inquiry: The Francis Report. London: DH.

Diabetes UK (2012). *Key Statistics on diabetes.* London: Diabetes UK. www.diabetes.org.uk/Documents/Reports/Diabetes-in-the-UK-2012.pdf (last accessed: 1 March 2013).

Jones, R. & Trigg, R. (2007). *Dementia and serious sight loss. Occasional Paper No 11.* London: Thomas Pocklington Trust.

Lievesley, N. (2010). *The Future Ageing of the Ethnic Minority Population of England and Wales.* London: Runnymede Trust/Centre for Policy on Ageing. www.runnymedetrust.org/publications/147/32.html (Last accessed: 26 November 2013).

Luengo-Fernandez, R., Leal, J. & Gray, A. (2010). *Dementia 2010: the economic burden of dementia and associated research funding in the United Kingdom.* Cambridge: Alzheimer's Research Trust. http://www.herc.ox.ac.uk/pubs/downloads/dementiafullreport (Last accessed: 6 May 2014).

Minassian, D. & Reidy, A. (2009). *Future Sight Loss UK 2: An epidemiological and economic model for sight loss in the decade 2010–2020.* London: EpiVision and Royal National Institute of Blind People.

Minassian, D.C., Reidy, A., Lightstone, A. & Desai, P. (2011). Modelling the prevalence of age-related macular degeneration (2010–2020) in the UK: expected impact of anti-vascular endothelial growth factor (VEGF) therapy. *British Journal of Ophthalmology.* doi: 10.1136/bjo. 2010. 195370.

Moriarty, J., Sharif, N. & Robinson, J. (2011). Black and minority ethnic people with dementia and their access to support and services. *Research Briefing* **35**. London: Social Care Institute for Excellence. www.scie.org.uk/publications/briefings/files/briefing35.pdf (Last accessed: 26 November 2013).

NICE (May 2008). Type 2 diabetes: the management of type 2 diabetes. http://guidance.nice.org.uk/CG66 (Last accessed: 19 March 2014).

NICE (May 2009). Type 2 diabetes: newer agents. www.nice.org.uk/nicemedia/live/12165/44318/44318.pdf (Last accessed: 19 March 2014).

NICE (2009). Glaucoma: diagnosis and management of chronic open-angle glaucoma and ocular hypertension. Clinical Guideline 85. London: NICE.

Nursing and Midwifery Council (2009). Guidance: for care of older people. London: NMC. www.nmc-uk.org documents/guidance/guidance-for-the-care-of-older-people.pdf (Last accessed: 19 March 2014).

Nyman, S.R., Gosney, M.A., & Victor, C.R. (2010). The psychosocial impact of vision loss on older people. *Generations Review.* **20**, 2 April.

Rovner, B.W., Casten, R.J., Hegel, M.T., Leiby, B.E. & Tasman, W.S. Preventing Depression in Age-Related Macular Degeneration (AMD) Trial (2007). *The Archives of General Psychiatry.* **64**, 886–92.

Royal College of Ophthalmologists (2010). *Cataract Surgery Guidelines.* September 2010. London: RCO.

Royal National Institute of Blind People (2009a). *Cost Oversight? The Cost of Eye Disease and Sight Loss in the UK Today and in the Future Report.* London: RNIB.
www.rnib.org.uk/getinvolved/campaign/policy/socialcare/reports/Pages/cost-oversight-report.aspx

Royal National Institute of Blind People (2009b). *Future Sight Loss UK (1): The Economic Impact of Partial Sight and Blindness in the UK Population.* Full report prepared by Access Economic Limited: London.

Royal National Institute of Blind People (2009c). Low Vision Service Outcomes: A Systematic Review. Low Vision Service Model Evaluation (LOVSME) Project. London: RNIB.

Royal National Institute of Blind People (2013a). *UK Vision Strategy 2013–2018 – Vision 2020 UK*.
www.vision2020uk.org.uk/ukvisionstrategy/core/core_picker/download.asp?id=539&filetitle=UK+Vision (Last accessed: 22 November 2013).

Royal National Institute of Blind People (2013b). 'Sight loss UK 2013. The latest evidence'.
www.rnib.org.uk/sites/default/files/Sight_loss_UK_2013_pdf (Last accessed: 19 April 2014).

Seewoodhary, R. & Watkinson, S. (2009). Treatment and management of ocular conditions in older people. *Nursing Standard.* **23** (35), 48–56.

Shahid, K.S. (2012). 'Visual Impairment: Understanding the Psychosocial Impact'. Paper presented at the 2012 American Academy of Optometry annual meeting. Phoenix, Arizona, US.

UK National Statistics Publication Hub (2014) Older People. Available at
http://www.statistics.gov.uk (Search term: 'older people'. Last accessed: 19 April 2014).

Watkinson, S. (2009a). Visual impairment in older people. *Nursing Older People.* **21** (8), 30–36.

Watkinson, S. (2009b). Management of visual impairment in older people: what can the nurse do? *Aging Health.* **5** (6), 821–32.

World Health Organisation (2007). *The Right to Sight Global Initiative for the Elimination of Avoidable Blindness Action Plan 2006–2011.* Geneva, Austria: WHO.

Chapter 2

Current perspectives on managing older people with cataracts

Susan Watkinson and Cecilia Awelewa

This chapter covers

- Introduction
- Overview of cataract formation
- Types of age-related cataract
- Current approaches to treatment
- Risks of cataract surgery
- Indications for cataract surgery
- Cataract care as day case surgery
- Pre-operative assessment
- Medical considerations
- Special investigations
- Types of intra-ocular lens
- Telephone assessment: pre- and post-cataract surgery
- Patient education
- Discharge planning
- The specialist ophthalmic nurse's role on the day of surgery
- The future role of the specialist ophthalmic nurse
- Future perspectives
- Conclusion

Introduction

This chapter considers current perspectives on managing the care of older people with cataracts on a day care surgery unit, and makes specific reference to the role of the specialist ophthalmic nurse (SON). As highlighted in Chapter 1, visual impairment can have a considerable impact on the quality of older people's lives. This is equally true of older people who develop cataract blindness. The chapter begins with an overview, covering the structure of the lens, the pathogenesis of cataract formation, the main types of cataract, the risk factors for cataract, and current approaches to treatment.

The importance and significance of pre-operative assessment and investigations will subsequently be discussed, with specific reference to the need for skilled biometry as a basis for an accurate dioptric power prescription of intra-ocular lenses. The operative procedure, together with potential post-operative complications, will be outlined. The role and responsibilities of the specialist ophthalmic nurse in managing older people with cataracts will be discussed in some detail. Again, as mentioned in Chapter 1, it is imperative that the ophthalmic nurse should be highly skilled and competent in delivering the latest technology, as this can make a big difference to the care and treatment outcomes experienced by the patient. Finally, future perspectives will be outlined, before concluding the chapter.

Overview of cataract formation

A cataract is opacity of the lens, causing it to become greyish-white in colour (Kanski & Bowling 2011). Figure 2.1 shows its typical appearance.

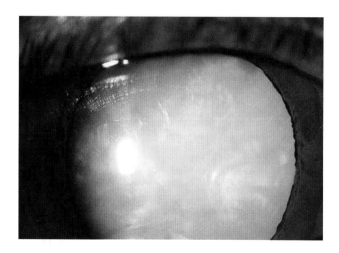

Figure 2.1: Typical appearance of a cataract

Cataract is an abnormal progressive condition. Risk factors include smoking, alcohol consumption, prolonged exposure to sunlight (specifically ultraviolet radiation), corticosteroid use, and medical conditions such as diabetes, cardiovascular disease and renal disease (Dhillon & Lascaratos 2009). Progressive cataract is also associated with poor health and poor life expectancy, and a history of poor nutrition and dehydration (Dhillon & Lascaratos 2009). However, most cataracts are linked to ageing. They usually occur bilaterally, although the rate of progression is seldom equal (James & Bron 2011). The signs and symptoms of a cataract are presented below.

Table 2.1: Signs and symptoms of a cataract

- Painless loss of vision
- White opacity through the pupil
- Gradual deterioration of sight
- Misty or cloudy vision
- Blurred images
- Sensitivity to light and glare
- Dimming of colours.

(Adapted from Kanski & Bowling 2011)

Structure of the lens

The lens is a biconvex, avascular, transparent structure, approximately 4mm thick and 9mm in diameter (Riordan-Eva & Whitcher 2008). It is suspended behind the iris by the suspensory ligament (zonule), which connects it to the ciliary body (see Figure 2.2, over page).

The zonule is composed of numerous fibrils, which arise from the surface of the ciliary body and insert into the lens equator. Aqueous humour is present in front of the lens, and posterior to it is vitreous humour.

The lens is composed of a nucleus and cortex, and lined by an anterior capsule (at the front) and a posterior capsule (at the back). The anterior lens capsule is a semi-permeable membrane, through which water and electrolytes may pass. The nucleus and cortex are made up of concentric lamellae; the nucleus is harder than the cortex (Riordan-Eva & Whitcher 2008).

The lens consists of about 65% water, about 35% protein, and a trace of minerals common to other body tissues. Potassium is more concentrated in the lens than in most tissues. Ascorbic acid and glutathione are present in both oxidised and reduced forms. There are no pain fibres, blood vessels or nerves in the lens (Riordan-Eva & Whitcher 2008).

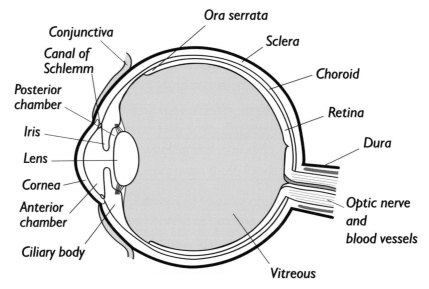

Figure 2.2: Diagram showing position of the lens

Pathogenesis

The transparency of the crystalline lens relies on a regular arrangement of the cells and fibres within the lining capsule (Dhillon & Lascaratos 2009). However, with age, sub-epithelial fibres are continually produced and added to the nucleus of the lens, which contains the oldest lens fibres. This means that the lens gradually becomes larger and less elastic throughout life (Riordan-Eva & Whitcher 2008, Dhillon & Lascaratos 2009). In addition, metabolic or biochemical insult may give rise to loss in fibre arrangement and transparency, resulting in a focal or diffuse opacity, which may have a measurable effect on vision.

Types of age-related cataract

There are three main types of age-related cataract:

1. Nuclear sclerosis: gradually deepening brunescence (see Figure 2.3)
2. Sub-capsular: shallow opacification just beneath the capsule, more commonly posterior than anterior (see Figure 2.4)
3. Cortical: discrete spoke-like opacities of the cortex (see Figure 2.5, page 28).

(Adapted from Batterbury et al. 2009)

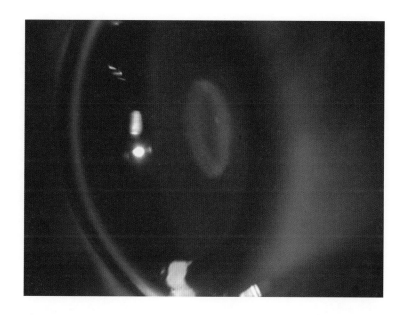

Figure 2.3: A nuclear cataract

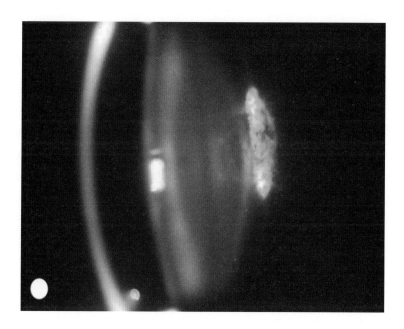

Figure 2.4: A posterior sub-capsular cataract

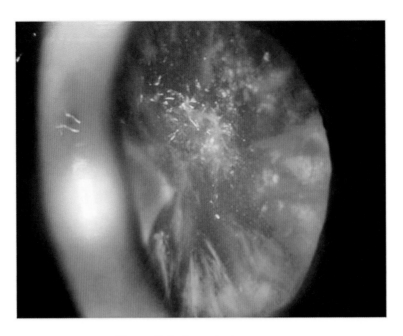

Figure 2.5: A cortical cataract

Risk factors for the above specific types of age-related cataract have been identified, based on anatomic morphology. For example, nuclear cataract is associated with smoking; posterior sub-capsular with diabetes and corticosteroids; and cortical cataract with ultraviolet light exposure (Dhillon & Lascaratos 2009).

Current approaches to treatment

Surgery is the only treatment for a cataract (Kanski & Bowling 2011) and is carried out as a day case procedure under local anaesthesia. Improvements in techniques of cataract removal, and correction of the resultant refractive error by inserting an intra-ocular lens implant (IOL), rank amongst the major medical advances of the last two decades (Batterbury *et al.* 2009). The benefits of such surgery lead to an improved quality of life and 80–90% of patients achieve 6/12 vision or better (Batterbury *et al.* 2009).

Phacoemulsification

Phacoemulsification is the current treatment of choice. This procedure involves removing the cataract, using a probe inserted through a small incision, and inserting a folded IOL implant. A transparent viscoelastic substance made of hyaluronic acid is first injected into the anterior chamber, providing the corneal endothelium with a protective layer. A disc of the anterior capsule is then peeled off the lens, allowing access to the lens nucleus and cortex. The probe ultrasonically fragments the lens nucleus into small particles (phacoemulsification), which are then removed through a suction device from the eye. A constant flow of saline cools the tip of the probe and helps to maintain the anterior chamber depth. After removal of the nucleus, residual cortex is aspirated from the eye. The implant is placed within the capsular bag (Batterbury et al. 2009).

Risks of cataract surgery

The vast majority of patients undergoing cataract surgery will have a successful outcome but there is still a risk of complications. Serious complications include choroidal haemorrhage and endophthalmitis (an aggressive intra-ocular infection) although this is extremely rare. Sight loss can also arise from a breach in the posterior capsule, macular oedema, or a failing corneal endothelium (Dhillon & Lascaratos 2009). In particular, myopic patients are at risk of retinal detachment when vitreous gel escapes from the eye through a torn posterior capsule. Diabetes predisposes individuals to macular oedema, and patients with shallow anterior chambers (associated with hypermetropia) may have a compromised 'dystrophy' affecting their corneal endothelium (Dhillon & Lascaratos 2009).

Indications for cataract surgery

In general, surgery is performed to improve visual outcome and restore quality of life. When activities of daily living (such as washing, dressing and cooking) become increasingly difficult for the older person to perform, due to impaired vision, surgery will need to be considered. The lifestyle needs that trigger referral to an eye surgeon often include difficulties in meeting the legal requirement for driving, misjudging distances and depths, problems recognising faces and bus numbers and reading computer displays, and frustration with the inability to pursue hobbies such as reading, gardening, travelling or sport (Dhillon & Lascaratos 2009).

Other indications include diabetic retinopathy, when the cataract prevents adequate retinal examination or laser treatment, and lens-induced glaucoma or uveitis (Batterbury et al. 2009).

Cataract care as day case surgery

Over the past decade, day case cataract surgery has increased remarkably, due to the redesigning of the cataract service, the implementation of best practice, and in most organisations, the introduction of advanced technology, modern anaesthesia, a streamlined process and improved organisational delivery without compromising care (RCO 2010).

In the UK, approximately 400,000 NHS cataract operations were performed in 2010 and 2011 (Health and Social Care Information Centre 2011). These technological advances have impacted on the role of the specialist ophthalmic nurse who has the responsibility of keeping up to date with professional knowledge and practice in order to manage the care of older patients with cataracts. The holistic approach adopted by specialist ophthalmic nurses throughout the UK has been remarkable in the areas of health promotion, informed consent, and accurate history-taking related to cardiovascular problems and diabetes, and recording blood pressure both pre-operatively and on the day of surgery. Adequate preparation is deemed to be essential in order to ensure positive outcomes for patients, surgeons and ophthalmic nurses.

Recent advances in a multidisciplinary approach to the day care cataract service have led to a dramatic reduction in the typical length of the older patient's stay in hospital – and consequently a higher patient satisfaction rate. Understandably, older people are much happier in their home environment. Providing accurate information for older patients undergoing surgery provided by the cataract day care service has also played a pivotal role in promoting their level of independence, reducing anxiety, improving morale and promoting patient empowerment (NMC 2008). Most issues are resolved at the pre-assessment stage. Providing a patient-focused service leads to considerable cost savings and reductions in the waiting list numbers. Figure 2.6 shows the current treatment pathway to the day care cataract service, which operates in all ophthalmic centres thoughout the UK.

> **1** Patient sees optometrist who makes provisional diagnosis and refers patient to hospital. GP is informed. Hospital books appointment date, and sends information to patient beforehand.

> **2** Patient visits hospital for confirmation of diagnosis by ophthalmologist and pre-op assessment. Both are done at the same visit.

> **3** Day of surgery (shorter stay in hospital).

> **4** Patient seen by nurse post-operatively; discharged if all is well; seen by ophthalmologist if any problems.

Figure 2.6: Current treatment pathway

This treatment pathway is implemented in many regions so that the optometrist has the power to refer patients. The primary care physician and the optometrist need to work in collaboration to ensure effective communication. At the second stage of this treatment pathway (see Table 2.2), it is important that older patients visit hospital for confirmation of their diagnosis and to ensure that they are assessed and deemed suitable for surgery. Conditions such as blepharitis, conjunctivitis and other eye infections may be detected and appropriately treated at this stage.

Following treatment of the condition, the patient will be booked for surgery and a pre-operative assessment will be undertaken.

Pre-operative assessment

The main objective of pre-operative assessment is to ensure that patients are fit for surgery, as indicated in the above treatment pathway, and a care plan is put in place to ensure improved surgical outcomes (RCO 2010). Walsgrove (2006) summarises the main aims of pre-operative assessment as follows (see Table 2.2).

Table 2.2: Main aims of pre-operative assessment

- To reduce patient risk to a minimum
- To identify patient suitability and/or fitness for surgery/anaesthesia
- To provide information for informed choices and consent
- To reduce fears and anxieties
- To help ensure better use of theatre and ward resources
- To improve the surgical patient's hospital experience.

(Adapted from Walsgrove 2006)

The role of the specialist ophthalmic nurse

The role of the SON in pre-operative assessment is that of an educator. Having assessed and acquired a sound knowledge of the older patient's condition, the procedure to be undertaken and the nurse's role in the process, the SON should offer support, reduce the patient's anxiety and promote confidence in the surgical team. In addition, the SON should help the older patient to prepare for surgery, and improve morale and promote patient empowerment – because the patient has a right to receive information about their condition

(NMC 2008). The SON must be a good communicator, as difficulties in communication can be a potential barrier to the process of pre-operative assessment. This means using simple language, avoiding medical jargon and allowing time for the patient to ask questions at any stage, supported by written information. Effective communication between patient and healthcare staff will enable any health organisation to meet the requirements of current government health policy (DH 2010).

The needs of older people

As a distinct age group, older people have specific problems, and their care must be tailored accordingly. The role of the SON is to identify their medical, physical and psychological needs, taking into consideration their lifestyle as well as ensuring that their privacy, dignity and confidentiality are maintained at all times (NMC 2008).

Often there are mobility problems due to strokes and fractured limbs as a result of falling. Older people therefore need to be supported in their movements, positioning and when walking around their environment (Hardy 2009). Physical disabilities, such as arthritis in the hands, will make it difficult to instil eye drops post-operatively. Older people should therefore be provided with the necessary guidance to facilitate their own eye drop instillation. Importantly, the older person's carer or family members should also be encouraged to provide continuity of care following surgery by being shown how to instil eye drops safely and accurately, since this is essential to promote healing and prevent complications.

Hearing difficulties, forgetfulness or cognitive impairment (such as mild dementia or mild depression) will impede the ability to communicate effectively. Other communication difficulties may arise due to overall anxiety, lack of confidence, and being in a strange environment. In the case of older people from ethnic minorities, language barriers may make communication problematic, causing additional anxiety and stress. To overcome some of the associated communication difficulties, it will be necessary to provide written information in the appropriate language as required, and according to local Trust policy.

Interpreting services must also be available both at the pre- and post-operative stages, as required. All the problems highlighted above need to be addressed at the pre-operative stage.

In general, the SON acts as a liaison officer between internal and external agencies, gathering information as well as implementing discharge planning. The SON should have a real influence on the quality, effectiveness and efficiency of the older patient's journey. A sound knowledge of clinical risk assessment is of paramount importance. Above all, the SON has a responsibility to help assess the older patient's suitability for surgery and identify the best choice of anaesthetic; and this must be a protocol-driven process. If the SON can effectively manage pre-assessment clinics during the pre-operative assessment stage, this will considerably reduce the number of cancelled cases on the day of surgery, thereby increasing patient throughput, which is at the heart of the government's agenda.

Medical considerations

General health evaluation

Pre-operative assessment entails a general health check of the patient, including, visual acuity, blood pressure, meticillin-resistant staphylococcus aureusis (MRSA) screening, current medications, allergies and blood sugar levels. If there are cardiac problems, an electrocardiogram (ECG) might also be necessary.

The SON requires good technical knowledge and skill in the use of the slit lamp to examine the eye when measuring intra-ocular pressure (IOP) and when performing biometry to select the intra-ocular lens for insertion and for the desired refractive result post-surgery. The pre-operative assessment period provides an opportunity to assess how the patient will manage at home with the instillation of eye drops and to demonstrate to the older person a safe and correct drop instillation technique. This will encourage older patients to take an active role in their own care.

Another crucially important issue is that of informed consent – that is, the patient's right to know and understand the procedure before agreeing and signing for it to be undertaken. Here, the role of the SON is paramount in ensuring that the older person has been provided with adequate information and understands the operative procedure to be performed. The older patient also needs to be psychologically prepared pre-operatively to reduce any fears and anxieties. The Royal College of Ophthalmologists (RCO 2010) makes it clear that it is the surgeon's responsibility to ensure that the patient has been given the appropriate information and that informed consent to surgery has been obtained and documented. Hence, the SON's role is crucial in making sure that all these safety checks are in place.

Patients taking anticoagulant therapy

The SON also plays a vital role in managing older patients who are receiving anticoagulant therapy. If this is not well managed, it can endanger the patient's health. Discontinuing anticoagulant therapy pre-operatively poses the risk of life-threatening complications such as death from cerebrovascular accident, transient ischaemic attack, myocardial infarction and pulmonary embolism (RCO 2010). Special care is therefore required for older patients on anticoagulant therapy who require cataract surgery. Fortunately, retrobulbar or peribulbar anaesthesia has been superseded by topical anaesthesia for cataract surgery, thereby averting the risk of retrobulbar and expulsive haemorrhages. In view of this, anticoagulant therapy should not pose any additional risk.

Warfarin is one of the anticoagulant tablets that is commonly used to reduce the incidence of life-threatening thromboembolic events in patients with cardiovascular conditions. The Royal College of Ophthalmologist Cataract Guidelines (2010) recommend that the international normalised ratio (INR) should be checked one week before surgery and then one day before surgery. It is recommended that the INR should be within the therapeutic ratio. The standard INR range for most clinical situations is 2–3.

The SON should liaise between the surgeon and the anaesthetist to agree on the appropriate regime before the commencement of surgery and this must be documented in the medical notes. Furthermore, there should be a local protocol in place to avoid cancellation on the day of surgery. A full explanation must be given to older patients as to what they need to do in order to avoid confusion and allay their anxieties. Currently, most patients on anticoagulant therapy are scheduled for local anaesthetic using topical gel to avoid the risk of sub-conjunctival or choroidal haemorrhage.

Special investigations

Biometry and keratometry investigations are performed to establish the correct lens implant to use during cataract surgery to meet the refractive needs of the individual patient (RCO 2010). Importantly, these investigations need to be performed well in advance of surgery to allow time for discussion between the SON, surgeon and patient to take place. This will ensure that the predictive refractive outcome is understood, and will also allow time for the correct intra-ocular lens to be ordered.

Essentially, there are two components of biometry investigation: axial length measurement (AL) by A-scan ultrasound or laser interferometry; and corneal curvature (K, K2) measurement by keratometry or corneal topography (RCO 2010). The SON plays a very important part in the care and use of the equipment required to perform biometry and obtain accurate biometrical data and interpretation of results.

Biometry

Biometry is the procedure used to measure the length and the thickness of the structures in the eye (AL measurement). Most ophthalmic departments prefer the use of Zeiss IOL Master, which is non-contact optical coherence interferometry. The equipment is easy to use. It involves placing the patient's chin on the chin rest and asking the patient to focus on the light for some minutes. The main aim of biometry is to allow the selection of an accurate IOL power in order to achieve the desired refractive result after cataract surgery, and this forms an essential part of the process. This investigation requires the specialist skills of the SON and the result is crucial to the success of the surgery.

Sometimes patients may require the services of an orthoptist, as some patients may develop diplopia due to asymmetrical cataract formation. Older patients with this problem will therefore require referral to the Orthoptic Department. An examination by the orthoptist at this stage may prove advantageous, as this may provide the first opportunity to identify the patient's problem. Since the orthoptist is a valuable member of the team undertaking biometry, this problem will be addressed at the same appointment. In some cases, cataract surgery tends to alleviate diplopia. However, some patients will experience diplopia after cataract surgery because of anisometropia. In this situation, cataract surgery on the second eye will need to be undertaken soon afterwards; for some patients, this will be within two weeks of their first eye cataract surgery.

Keratometry

This is the process of measuring the curvature of the cornea. The keratometer is a calibrated instrument that measures the radius of curvature of the cornea in two meridians 90 degrees apart. If the cornea is not perfectly spherical, the two radii will be different. This is known as astigmatism and is quantified by measuring the difference between the two radii of curvature (Riordan-Eva & Whitcher 2008). The process can be manual or automated with an average of three readings, but the automated process is quite common.

Biometry readings: 96% of axial length readings fall within the range of 21.0mm to 25.5mm; and for 60% of axial lengths it is between 22.5 and 24.5mm (RCO 2010). With reference to corneal curvature, 98% of K-readings fall within the range of 40 to 48D and 68% of K-readings are between 42 and 45D.

Overall, most individuals have similar axial lengths in each eye, except in the presence of certain pathological conditions such as unilateral refractive error, coloboma or staphyloma, which may affect eye size (RCO 2010). Equally, most corneas are regularly curved and similar between the two eyes. Any intra-ocular differences in axial length of more than 0.3mm, or K-readings that vary by more than 1 dioptre require confirmation. These results should only be accepted when repeated measurements show consistent results (RCO 2010). In the case of highly myopic eyes (axial length > 28mm), a B-scan should be performed to determine the presence of staphyloma (RCO 2010).

Types of intra-ocular lens

The main types of intra-ocular lenses inserted during cataract surgery are summarised below and in Figure 2.7. Some intra-ocular lenses are foldable and others are non-foldable. The foldable ones are made of materials such as silicon and acrylic; the non-foldable lenses are made from PMMA (that is, hard plastic materials).

● Phakic IOLS: This type of lens is used for myopic and hyper-myopic patients.

● Phakic Toric IOLS: These are best for patients with a significant astigmatism, and they will improve the patient's distance vision without glasses.

● Non-Phakic Monofocal IOLS: These may reduce a patient's need for glasses after surgery.

● Non-Phakic Multifocal IOLS: These are best for patients who desire both good distance and reading vision without glasses.

● Non-Phakic Accommodative IOLs: These are best for patients whose choice is for uncorrected distance and intermediate vision and who find it acceptable to wear glasses for extended periods of reading.

However, special powers or models of IOL may be required for some older patients and these may have to be specially ordered. Whatever the choice of IOL, the surgeon must discuss and gain the consent of the patient so the role of the SON is crucial.

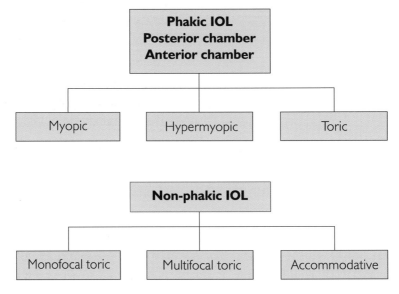

Figure 2.7: A summary of the main types of intra-ocular lenses inserted during cataract surgery

Telephone assessment: pre- and post-cataract surgery

Due to the recent increase in older patients waiting for second eye cataract surgery, together with staff shortages and lack of space in most ophthalmic departments, it has become more difficult to arrange a second visit. It has therefore been suggested that a post-cataract surgery telephone assessment could replace a further visit. In the past, it was seen as good practice to telephone patients on the first post-operative day to assess their condition and progress. However, most ophthalmic departments have now phased out this approach, especially where surgery is uncomplicated and provided there is a mechanism in place for the older patient to contact the hospital in the event of encountering any problems related to the eye. The current protocol is that second eye operation dates are booked at the patient's first post-operative appointment visit. The SON in charge of the clinic will arrange for the patient to be telephone-assessed and a date will be given, provided the criteria are met (RCO 2010). However, this process has to be managed effectively to ensure that crucial issues are not overlooked, which could subsequently lead to cancellation on the day of surgery.

Patient education

The role of the SON in providing patient education about ocular health is vital (RCN 2012). The Royal College of Nursing also recognises that the SON has to give the patient the relevant information in order to gain understanding and confidence. Providing accurate information, both verbal and written, is crucial, as this will facilitate the older person's compliance with pre- and post-operative treatment and the protocol for surgery.

Information must be given about the surgery, duration of stay in hospital, fasting instructions, time of arrival, possible time of discharge and prescribed medication following surgery. The role of the SON in health promotion and health education for older patients and their families is of paramount importance. The older patient and family members must be shown how to instil eye drops correctly and safely, and how to clean the eyelids daily as part of good eye care to prevent infection. Information must also be provided about the importance of daily observation of the eyes to check for any signs of infection.

Discharge planning

Ideally discharge planning should start at the pre-operative assessment stage. All social aspects and the well-being of the patient should be assessed and documented during this period. This will include:

● Booking transport for those who meet the criteria

- Contacting social services if the need arises
- Arranging for other community care services, or arranging a district nurse or primary care physician
- Making arrangements for all eye drops to be dispensed by the pharmacy.

Dealing with all these issues will help to facilitate a smooth discharge home, and lead to quick recovery and a high level of patient satisfaction.

The specialist ophthalmic nurse's role on the day of surgery

The SON needs to be adequately skilled and knowledgeable in order to meet the needs of the older patient both pre- and post-operatively (RCN 2009). Interpersonal skills are crucial in providing a welcoming environment, and showing concern for both older patients and their families will help to reduce stress and anxiety. As a competent practitioner, the SON must be willing to provide adequate information to allay any fears and anxieties about the forthcoming surgery, and, above all, compassion must be shown towards older patients at every stage (DH 2012). The ability to assess, plan and implement individual care using a holistic approach, and maintain confidentiality, privacy and dignity, must be demonstrated as per the locally agreed protocol and guidelines.

The specialist ophthalmic nurse in the operating theatre

The SON's role in the operating theatre is that of a technical expert, requiring familiarity with all the equipment. Good rapport must be maintained between the operating surgeon and the scrub nurse for a successful surgical outcome. A sound knowledge of ophthalmic instruments, drugs and drops is essential. In most ophthalmic settings in the UK, the operating theatre nurse (as opposed to the surgeon) takes on the role of draping the patient. The whole team takes responsibility for infection control; hence every team member must work to the agreed protocol and be regularly monitored in order to reduce the risk of infection to the minimum. The operating theatre staff must have all the expertise needed to deal with each stage of the surgery. In other words, the operating department assistant must make sure that all patient's details are checked, all monitoring is checked and recorded, and the operating eye duly signed for and marked to prevent any mistakes. Ideally, the anaesthetist should be present. Where this is not possible, a highly qualified theatre SON with advanced life support skills and equipment must be present. For a successful surgical outcome, the rule of sterility must be observed throughout, while fulfilling government expectations on efficiency, effectiveness and improved performance targets.

The future role of the specialist ophthalmic nurse

In summary, the future role of the SON will be to continue to advance professional knowledge and practice to maintain and improve older patients' ocular health. This will also involve collaborating with other healthcare professionals in order to make a difference to the quality of life of older patients.

The SON's commitment to continuous self-education, research and the development of critical thinking skills will enhance ophthalmic practice in the future (Watkinson 2009). Research awareness will enable more effective delivery of care using an evidence base to meet the needs of the older patient and implement change (Marsden 2008). Moreover, being highly innovative in practice is one of the key targets to be achieved by healthcare professionals in the NHS as a means of increasing efficiency and productivity (DH 2012).

The SON will be expected to demonstrate effective use of critical appraisal skills to assess and implement new research evidence, where appropriate, to advance ophthalmic practice for the benefit of older patients with visual impairment (Watkinson 2009). Delivery of high-quality care and the ability to demonstrate initiative and innovation in practice to increase efficiency and productivity will be key challenges for the future (DH 2012).

Future perspectives

In the future, phacoemulsification as a surgical technique is likely to be replaced by femtosecond laser-assisted refractive surgery. It is predicted that this major advance in ophthalmic surgery will become part of mainstream, commonly used technology in advanced countries by 2020 (Lindstrom 2011).

Femtosecond lasers emit extremely short optical impulses, as short as one-quadrillionth of a second ($1.0 \times 10\text{-}15$ seconds). With such ultra-short pulses, tissue can be cut more precisely and with practically no heat development. The femtosecond laser is therefore a highly accurate surgical laser, which can be used in high-precision ocular microsurgery (Moshirfar et al. 2011). This approach offers a much higher level of accuracy and predictability than current cataract surgery by phacoemulsification (using ultrasound technology) and could potentially make the procedure even safer, with visual outcomes to match patient needs.

Advantages and disadvantages of laser-assisted surgery

Advantages include firstly a reduced risk of intraoperative complications, especially in more complicated forms of cataract. Secondly, the laser system allows for highly accurate positioning and concentration of the artificial intra-ocular lens, thus reducing optical aberrations and refractive errors (Lindstrom 2011).

One disadvantage associated with laser cataract surgery is the risk of elevated intra-ocular pressure (IOP) and the potential for IOP-related complications in older people with cataracts (Schultz 2013). In addition to increasing IOP as a result of the application of the vacuum ring and laser-patient docking station, femtosecond laser treatment leads to the production of plasma and expanding cavitation bubbles in the anterior chamber (Shultz 2013). The level of increase in IOP induced by the docking device has not yet been adequately quantified in published studies. Nevertheless, this may become a significant contraindication for patients with glaucoma, optic neuropathies, or borderline endothelial pathology for the future (Moshirfar *et al.* 2011).

However, the most controversial aspect will be the issue of funding this new and expensive technology and assessing its financial feasibility in the current context of economic strictures. These laser machines with integrated OCT or Scheimpflug technology will add considerable expense to the current procedure. Undoubtedly, the issue of cost will be the subject of ongoing debate.

Conclusion

In summary, this chapter has considered in some detail current perspectives on managing the care of older people undergoing cataract surgery on a day care surgery unit. An overview of this condition was initially presented with reference to risk factors, signs and symptoms, pathogenesis, types of senile cataract, current approaches to treatment, the risks of surgery, and the main indications for cataract surgery.

The concept of cataract care as day surgery was considered, before discussing the role and responsibilities of the specialist ophthalmic nurse during the pre-assessment stage and the special investigations undertaken, the pre-operative, operative and post-operative stages, and discharge planning stage. From this discussion, it emerged that the specialist ophthalmic nurse must continue to advance professional knowledge and practice to help maintain and improve the older patient's ocular health and increase the delivery of high-quality care in the midst of many challenges. Importantly, the ophthalmic nurse must remain highly skilled and competent in delivering the latest technology but, above all, demonstrate compassionate care to older people undergoing cataract surgery.

Finally, future perspectives on ophthalmic surgery were outlined, particularly the exciting prospect of femtosecond laser-assisted refractive cataract surgery becoming mainstream technology by 2020 and revolutionising cataract surgery. In the next chapter, age-related macular degeneration (a major ocular disease affecting older people) will be presented and discussed.

References

Batterbury, M., Bowling, B. & Murphy, C. (2009). *Ophthalmology. An Illustrated Colour Text.* 3rd edn. Edinburgh: Elsevier Churchill Livingstone.

Department of Health (2010). *Equity and excellence. Liberating the NHS.* London: DH.

Department of Health (2012). *Compassion in Practice. Nursing, Midwifery and Care Staff. Our Vision and Strategy.* London: DH.

Dhillon, B. & Lascaratos, G. (2009). Age-related vision loss: cataract. *Ageing Health.* **5** (6), 813–19.

Hardy, J. (2009). Supporting patients undergoing cataract extraction surgery. *Nursing Standard.* **24** (14), 51–6.

Health and Social Care Information Centre (2001). Hospital Episode Statistics: Inpatient headline summary. 2010/2011. HSCIC. www.hesonline.nhs.uk (last accessed: 20 July 2013).

James, B. & Bron, A. (2011). *Lecture Notes on Ophthalmology.* 11th edn. Oxford: Wiley Blackwell.

Kanski, J. & Bowling, B. (2011). *Clinical Ophthalmology: A Systematic Approach.* 7th edn. London: Elsevier.

Lindstrom, R.L. (2011). The Future of Laser-assisted Refractive Cataract Surgery. *Journal of Refractive Surgery.* August 27 (8), 552–3.

Marsden, J. (2008). *An Evidence Base for Ophthalmic Nursing Practice.* Oxford: Wiley.

Moshirfar, M., Churgin, D.S. & Hsu, M. (2011). Femtosecond Laser-Assisted Cataract Surgery: A Current Review. *Middle East African Journal of Ophthalmology.* Oct–Dec. **18** (4), 285–91.

Nursing and Midwifery Council (2008). The Code: Standards of Conduct, Performance and Ethics for Nurses and Midwives. London: NMC. www.nmc-uk.org/Documents/Standards/The-code-A4-20100406.pdf (Last accessed: 20 April 2014).

Riordan-Eva, P. & Whitcher, J. (2008). *Vaughan and Asbury's General Ophthalmology.* 17th edn. New York NY: Lange Medical Books/McGraw-Hill.

Royal College of Nursing (2009). *The Nature, Scope and Value of Ophthalmic Nursing.* 3rd edn. London: Royal College of Nursing.

Royal College of Nursing (2012). *Ophthalmic Nursing: An integrated career and competence framework.* London: RCN.

Royal College of Ophthalmologists (2010). *Cataract Surgery Guidelines.* London: RCO.

Schultz, M.C. (2013). Update on Laser Cataract Surgery. *Cataract and Refractive Surgery Today Europe.* March 63–5.

Walsgrove, H. (2006). Putting education into practice for pre-operative patient assessment. *Nursing Standard.* **20** (47), 35–9.

Watkinson, S. (ed). (2009). *Issues in Ophthalmic Practice: Current and future challenges.* Keswick, Cumbria: M&K Publishing.

Chapter 3

Managing the care of older people with age-related macular degeneration

Susan Watkinson

This chapter covers

- Introduction
- Changes associated with age-related macular degeneration (AMD)
- Pathogenesis
- Classification and clinical features
- Aetiology
- Diagnosing AMD
- Treatment – current and future perspectives
- Managing older people with AMD – the role of the health and social care professional
- Managing older patients undergoing intra-vitreal therapy
- Future perspectives on AMD
- Conclusion

Introduction

This chapter considers the management of older people with dry and wet age-related macular degeneration (AMD). Initially, it provides an overview of the physiological changes that occur in the ageing macula. It also describes the pathogenesis, classification, clinical features, aetiology, and current and future perspectives on the treatment of the condition, with reference to research evidence.

The health and social care professional's role in the clinical management of AMD is discussed, with specific focus on managing older people undergoing intra-vitreal therapy. Health education, effective communication and counselling skills are highlighted as key elements in caring for and supporting older people who are adjusting to the shock of visual loss and its effects on their quality of life. The management of Charles Bonnet Syndrome is also discussed, as it is one of the most frightening conditions associated with visual loss.

The chapter concludes with a consideration of some future perspectives on the role of the health and social care professional, with reference to the predicted increase in the number of older people likely to encounter this irreversible eye disease.

Changes associated with age-related macular degeneration (AMD)

Age-related macular degeneration (AMD) is the term applied to ageing changes that occur, without an obvious cause, in the macula, the central area of the retina, in people aged 50 years and above (RCO 2009). Its prevalence increases after the age of 75 (RCO 2009) and it is the leading cause of irreversible blindness in people aged over 50 in the western world (Congdon et al. 2004). In the United Kingdom, AMD accounts for half of all registered blindness (Bunce & Wormald 2008). Given the predicted increase in the ageing population as a result of demographic changes over the coming years, the incidence of age-related macular degeneration will continue to rise (NICE 2008).

The macula is the most sensitive area of the retina and is 5.5–6mm in diameter. Vision is sharpest in the fovea, the central area, which is 0.25mm in diameter, is the narrowest part of the retina and contains only cone cells. Cone cells are responsible for daylight vision and for detecting colours (Marsden 2006). Overall, the macula provides fine visual discrimination, optimal visual acuity and colour vision (Riordan-Eva & Whitcher 2008).

Any deterioration of the macula will therefore affect central vision. Figure 3.1 shows a healthy retina with a normal macula, and normal blood vessels entering and leaving at the optic disc. Figure 3.2 shows degenerative changes occurring in the macula caused by choroidal neovascularisation. Figure 3.3 (page 46) provides a schematic diagram of the process of choroidal neovascularisation and the anatomical layers involved.

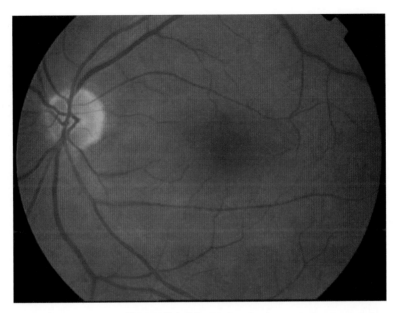

Figure 3.1: Normal macula

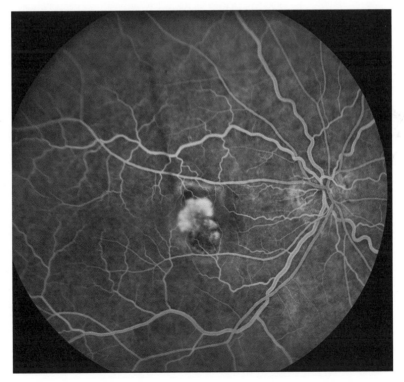

*Figure 3.2: An abnormal macula showing degenerative changes
caused by choroidal neovascularisation*

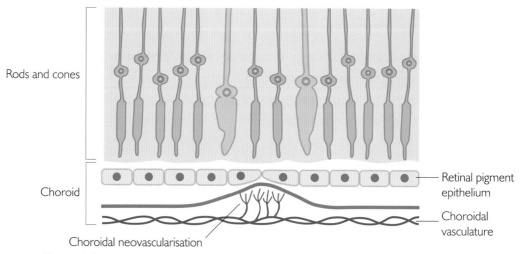

Rods and cones

Choroid

Retinal pigment epithelium

Choroidal vasculature

Choroidal neovascularisation

Figure 3.3: A schematic diagram of the process of choroidal neovascularisation

Pathogenesis

The pathogenesis of AMD is poorly understood. However, degeneration of the retinal pigment epithelium, changes in Bruch's membrane and the formation of sub-retinal deposits (drusen) are central to progression of the disease (Riordan-Eva & Whitcher 2008). Bruch's membrane is the innermost layer of the choroid. It consists of five layers and its innermost layer forms the basement membrane of the retinal pigment epithelium in the retina. Figure 3.4 shows its anatomical position.

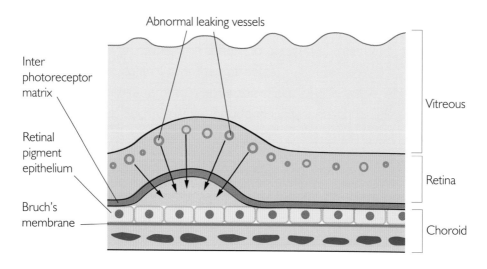

Abnormal leaking vessels

Inter photoreceptor matrix

Retinal pigment epithelium

Bruch's membrane

Vitreous

Retina

Choroid

Figure 3.4: Anatomical position of Bruch's membrane

The inter photoreceptor matrix fills that part of the eye known as the sub-retinal space. It is located between the outer limiting membrane of the retina and the border of the retinal pigment epithelium (RPE). It is a unique matrix that surrounds the photoreceptor inner and outer segments projecting from the outer retinal surface.

Progressive diffuse thickening of Bruch's membrane reduces the ability of oxygen to diffuse through to the retinal pigment epithelium and photoreceptors, leading to hypoxia. The latter gives rise to the release of growth factors, which stimulate the growth of new choroidal blood vessels. These vessels leak serous fluid or blood, resulting in distortion and reduced clarity of central vision (Riordan-Eva & Whitcher 2008).

Classification and clinical features

NICE (2008) classifies AMD as either 'dry' (non-exudative or non-neovascular) or 'wet' (exudative or neovascular). Table 3.1 (below) lists the signs and symptoms.

Table 3.1: Signs and symptoms of AMD

- Objects appear to change shape, size or colour
- Objects can appear to move or disappear
- Vision is centrally blurred
- Lines can appear distorted and/or wavy
- Dark spots can appear in central vision
- An area of blindness can block out several words at normal reading distance
- Difficulty seeing objects in bright sunlight
- Glare.

(Adapted from Kanski & Bowling 2011)

Dry AMD

Dry AMD is the most common form of AMD, usually with an insidious onset and rate of progression (Kanski & Bowling 2011). Visual loss results from a progressive degenerative process, which leads to cell death and atrophy of the retinal pigment epithelium (Riordan-Eva & Whitcher 2008). The retinal pigment epithelium that nourishes the macula and removes its metabolic waste starts to age and become less efficient, allowing fatty, yellow, metabolic waste products, known as drusen, to accumulate in the retina (Kanski & Bowling 2011).

The cells in the macula break down, causing central loss of vision but leaving peripheral vision unaffected (Kanski & Bowling 2011). This form accounts for 85% of cases of people with AMD and leads to a mild to moderate loss of sight (Kanski & Bowling 2011).

Over time, it can cause profound vision loss. Currently, there is no treatment for dry AMD (Kanski & Bowling 2011). Table 3.2 lists the specific signs and symptoms of this condition.

Table 3.2: Specific signs and symptoms of dry AMD

- Soft drusen may be present
- There are areas of increased pigment or hyperpigmentation (in the outer retina or choroid)
- There are areas of depigmentation or hypopigmentation of the retinal pigment epithelium
- The central vision deteriorates (when the atrophy is bilateral and involves the macula of both eyes)
- There is difficulty in reading, initially with smaller sizes of print and later with larger print.

Wet AMD

This type of AMD is less common, but it is increasing along with the size of the ageing population. Because of its aggressive nature, it can lead to severe sight loss in weeks or even days (Kanski & Bowling 2011), and accounts for 80 to 90% of all registered blind patients with AMD (Congdon et al. 2004).

Progressive diffuse thickening of Bruch's membrane reduces the ability of oxygen to diffuse through to the retinal pigment epithelium and photoreceptors, leading to local hypoxia. The latter gives rise to the release of growth factors and cytokines, which stimulate the growth of new choroidal blood vessels. These vessels leak serous fluid or blood into the macula, resulting in distortion and reduced clarity of central vision (Riordan-Eva and Whitcher, 2008). Peripheral vision is, however, retained.

Choroidal neovascularisation (CNV) can be subdivided into classic and occult forms according to its appearance on investigation by fluorescein angiography. The main difference between the two is that the classic form (leaking) is associated with a more abrupt and rapid progression of visual loss than the occult (quiescent) form (NICE 2008). In the advanced stages of wet AMD, CNV is commonly associated with permanent fibrous scarring of the macula (Wong et al. 2008). Table 3.3 lists the specific symptoms of wet AMD.

Table 3.3: Specific symptoms of wet AMD

Symptom	Description
General	Clouding, flickering, flashing lights, hallucinatory forms
Metamorphopsia	Central vision distorted – straight lines appearing bent
Scotoma	A blind spot in the visual field
Less visual acuity	Poorer ability to distinguish between letters such as 'o' and 'c'
Less contrast sensitivity	Poorer ability to distinguish between, for example, individual steps when going up and down stairs
Less colour vision.	Poorer ability to see colours.

(Adapted from Bressler 2002)

Aetiology

The exact aetiology of AMD is unknown, but age seems to be the risk factor that is most strongly associated with the condition (Chopdar et al. 2003). Other risk factors are listed in Table 3.4 (below).

Table 3.4: General and ocular risk factors associated with AMD

General factors	Ocular factors
• Smoking • Elevated cholesterol • Hypertension • Cardiovascular disease • Race – Caucasians are more likely to have choroidal neovascularisation • Family history of AMD.	• Presence of soft drusen • Macular pigmentary change • Choroidal neovascularisation in the other eye.

(Adapted from Chopdar et al. 2003)

The risk of developing AMD is 3.6 times greater for current and former smokers than for those who have never smoked (NICE 2008). Diet and nutrition may also play an important part in maintaining eye health. Treatment with oral vitamins and copper have been found to reduce the five-year risk of progression to late AMD (Riordan-Eva & Whitcher 2008).

Bosely (2009) has reported that the administration of an antioxidant supplement (containing vitamins C and E, zinc, and the carotenoids lutein and zeaxanthin) to a group of 400 people with AMD in one eye, and at risk of sight loss in the other eye, slowed the degeneration and sharpened their vision.

Virtually all studies to date have been designed to examine the effect of supplements on end-stage AMD. However, the evidence suggests that nutritional supplements have little or no effect in the primary prevention of early AMD (Chong et al. 2007). Reported evidence from a systematic review and meta-analysis suggest that vitamins A, C and E, zinc, lutein, zeaxanthin, alphacarotene and betacarotene, cryptoxanthin and lycopene have little or no effect in the primary prevention of early AMD (Chong et al. 2007). Further evidence from a systematic review of three randomised controlled trials also showed that antioxidant supplements did not prevent early AMD (Chong et al. 2007). Excessive sun exposure has been highlighted as a possible risk factor, but, as yet, this is unsupported by published studies (Khan et al. 2006).

Diagnosing AMD

An Amsler grid (AMD 2010) is a useful tool for diagnosing AMD, enabling patients to assess their own vision at home on a weekly basis. It also alerts the patient to any change or worsening of the condition. However, diagnosis is mainly based on an ophthalmoscopic examination using stereoscopic slit-lamp biomicroscopy with fundal examination, optical coherence tomography and fluorescein dye angiography. Optical coherence tomography is an advanced, non-invasive procedure that produces high-resolution, cross-sectional imaging of the retinal layers (Riordan-Eva & Whitcher 2008). Posterior segment optical coherence tomography enables a detailed analysis of the optic disc, retinal nerve fibre layer and macula. Microscopic changes in the macula can be imaged and measured (Riordan-Eva & Whitcher 2008).

Treatment – current and future perspectives
Dry AMD

No therapies are actually available for dry (atrophic) AMD, despite some experimental new pharmacological approaches (Querques et al. 2011). Huang et al. (2008) reported that people with dry AMD, who were at high risk of developing advanced AMD, lowered their risk by about 25% when treated with a high-dose combination of vitamin C, vitamin E, betacarotene and zinc. In this same high-risk group, these nutrients reduced the risk of vision loss caused by advanced AMD by about 19%. However, for those study participants who had either no AMD, or early AMD, the nutrients did not appear to provide any benefit.

Observational studies have also suggested benefits from increased dietary intake of macular xanthophylls and omega-3 fatty acids (Radu et al. 2005). Fenretinide, a hydrophobic drug structurally derived from vitamin A, reduces lipofuscin deposition interfering with fluorophores, vitamin A transport proteins, which seem to contribute directly to the pathogenesis of AMD (Radu et al. 2005). Fenretinide has produced positive results for slowing the progression of dry macular degeneration (National Institutes of Health 2007). Evidence suggests that oxidative stress and inflammation are linked to the progression of dry AMD. Topical use of OT-551, a patented small molecule that acts on oxidative stress and disease-induced inflammation, has been shown to be well tolerated by patients with dry AMD, and has not been associated with any serious adverse effects (Tanito et al. 2010). Nevertheless, in its current concentration and mode of delivery, OT-551 may be of limited or no benefit in treating dry AMD, since it has no significant effects on other outcomes (Wong et al. 2010).

Although there is no treatment for dry AMD that is currently approved by health authorities, older patients require regular monitoring because dry AMD can convert without warning to the wet form (Kanski & Bowling 2011). The provision of support and access to appropriate services and resources will be essential as part of their continuing care and management in the community, which will be addressed subsequently in this chapter.

Wet AMD

Overall, there is no cure for AMD. Previous management of wet AMD with laser or photodynamic therapy could at best stabilise or improve visual acuity in less than 10% of cases. However, new agents can target the bioactivity of vascular endothelial growth factor (VEGF) and have been reported to produce significant improvement in visual acuity in 40% of cases (CATT Research Group 2011).

For some time, the drugs of choice have been ranibizumab and bevacizumab. A key point here was the major difference in the cost of the two treatments. Ranibizumab was specifically engineered for ophthalmic use, whereas bevacizumab was designed for gastrointestinal cancer but appeared to work equally well in the eye. The current cost difference is £900 versus £50 per injection respectively. Bevacizumab, although not licensed, is used because it is cost-effective. These two drugs are antibodies, which target and neutralise VEGF. Bevacizumab is a potent inducer of vascular permeability and stimulator of angiogenesis, and may also have pro-inflammatory effects. All these factors are thought to affect the progression of wet AMD (NICE 2008).

These drugs are injected into the vitreous and specifically bind to and inhibit the VEGF. The procedure involves inserting the needle of the syringe containing the intra-vitreal drug perpendicular through the sclera, with the tip aimed towards the centre of the globe, to avoid any contact with the posterior lens. An appropriate volume (0.05–00.1ml) of the therapeutic agent is injected slowly and carefully, and the needle removed slowly (RCO 2009).

After the injection, it is important to check that the patient can count fingers or see hand movements to ensure that the central retinal artery is perfused (RCO 2009). There is good evidence that these new intra-vitreal injection therapies are effective and safe (Querques et al. 2011). Systematic reviews conclude that the prognosis for neovascular AMD is improved by clinical use of anti-VEGF drugs that target all isotypes of VEGF and maintain vision in over 90% and substantial improvement in 25–40% of patients (Takeda et al. 2007, Schmidt-Erfurth et al. 2007).

A monthly intra-vitreal injection of ranibizumab has been shown to be superior to placebo and photodynamic therapy in minimally classic and occult subtypes of neovascular AMD (Rosenfeld et al. 2006, Brown et al. 2009). Multiple ranibizumab injections are deemed safe over the long term for treating choroidal neovascularisation in AMD as this drug is well tolerated, and the incidence of serious adverse effects is low and unrelated to dose (Singer 2009, Boyer et al. 2009).

Nevertheless, the need for repeated intra-vitreal injections is a key limitation, with the associated potential risks of bacterial endophthalmitis, uveitis, retinal detachment and traumatic cataract (RCO 2009). To overcome this, combination treatments have been tried. These appear to reduce the need for retreatment, but visual results have not been as good as those recorded with ranibizumab alone.

Latest treatment for wet AMD

In October 2013, NICE approved the use of another drug, aflibercept, to rival ranibizumab (Lucentis). Although it costs the same as ranibizumab (Lucentis), it requires fewer injections, thus making it a more cost-effective treatment over time.

Aflibercept solution is recommended as an option for treating AMD only if:

- It is used in accordance with the recommendations for ranibizumab in the NICE technology appraisal guidance 155 (May 2012)
- The manufacturer provides aflibercept solution for injection with the discount agreed in the patient access scheme (NICE 2013).

Aflibercept solution for injection is a soluble vascular endothelial growth factor receptor fusion protein that binds to all forms of VEGF-A, VEGF-B, and the placental growth factor, thus preventing these factors from stimulating the growth of the fragile and permeable new blood vessels associated with wet AMD (NICE 2013).

The treatment should be given monthly for three consecutive 2mg doses, followed by one injection every two months, with each 100 microlitre vial containing 4mg of aflibercept. Aflibercept solution for injection must only be administered by a qualified doctor, experienced in administering intra-vitreal injections. There is no need for monitoring between injections. After the first 12 months, the treatment interval may be extended, based on visual and anatomic outcomes (NICE 2013).

Combination therapy

Combination therapy is likely to play an increasing role in treating wet AMD, and may improve visual acuity outcomes, reduce retreatment rates, and consequently extend treatment-free intervals (Patel 2009). Combination with photodynamic therapy seems to reduce the number of injections and to maintain the effects of treatment for longer (Chen et al. 2010). This may lead to a lower treatment burden for many patients and a reduction in overall cost of treatment. Numerous new drugs are being investigated, suggesting that new combinations will emerge.

Stem cell therapy

Currently, the use of stem cell therapy is under scrutiny regarding its role and efficacy in treating patients with AMD. Stem cell therapy is advantageous in that it replaces the damaged or dead retinal pigment epithelium and photoreceptor cells with viable cells. It can offer an unlimited supply of retinal precursors for endogenous repair and exogenous cell replacement. However, debate continues as to which type of stem cell is most appropriate for treating AMD. The types being considered are: adult-derived progenitor stem cells (including progenitor cells from ocular tissues), hematopoietic stem cells, embryonic stem cells, and induced pluripotent stem cells (Mooney & Lamotte 2011).

Encouragingly, stem cell therapy provides the potential to supply functioning cells, but clearly it is more complex to accomplish this and at the same time restore vision to AMD patients (Mooney & Lamotte 2011). In preliminary human pilot projects, stem cell therapy has shown promise in restoring some visual function to AMD patients. Nevertheless, several questions remain: What type of stem cell is best suited to treating AMD patients? How much visual function can be restored? Are the visual acuity improvements sustainable? Will stem cell therapy prove safe and effective? How might stem cells be used to restore function to higher visual pathways?

Managing older people with AMD – the role of the health and social care professional

Counselling and psychological support

Visual impairment is an important aspect of chronic illness and a cause of disability, which has a direct effect on physical function and performance (Hayman *et al.* 2007). Systematic reviews provide evidence of the effect of AMD on quality of life, which includes functional impairment, depression, anxiety and emotional distress (Berman & Brodaty 2006, Mitchell & Bradley 2006). Understandably, feelings of hopelessness, anxiety, depression and thoughts of suicide are often expressed by patients with AMD (Lewis & Southall 2006). Gaining insight into the patient's fears of going blind is therefore integral to the nurse's role. Counselling skills, active listening and positive responding are crucial to the delivery of quality care. Patients should be allowed to explore their feelings and thoughts as a basis for participation in their own care and future self-empowerment (Watkinson & Scott 2010).

Although dry AMD is slowly progressive and does not usually lead to vision loss, the loss of central vision can substantially reduce the patient's ability to function and self-care. Here, the health and social care professional's role is to provide reassurance and education on the use of low-vision aids to promote independence and self-care. Clinical follow-up is also beneficial to promote patient well-being and to rule out other age-associated eye pathologies such as glaucoma.

Wet AMD can progress rapidly and patients undergoing photodynamic therapy or intra-vitreal therapy (IVT) are likely to be anxious and apprehensive. On average, patients with wet AMD are almost twice as likely to be depressed as people with normal vision; and as the severity of the AMD increases, the patient's feelings of depression also increase (Creuss *et al.* 2006).

Spending quality time with the older patient is essential in order to explain the treatment and allay associated fears and anxieties (Watkinson 2010). Counselling skills are important in helping patients deal with the shock of visual loss and in providing the basis for their subsequent empowerment (Watkinson 2010). A quiet environment is essential for breaking bad news to older patients newly diagnosed with wet AMD. Older people require explanation and reassurance about the importance of treatment, treatment options and why, for example, the IVT procedure is appropriate for them. In some cases, support is also required when the patient has not met the criteria for commencing treatment. Explanation of what the procedure involves, what to expect and the associated possible complications of IVT is also important (Watkinson 2010). Clinical management of older patients undergoing IVT will be discussed later in this chapter.

Charles Bonnet syndrome (CBS)

In patients with moderate visual loss, approximately 10% will, at some point, experience visual hallucinations, a condition known as Charles Bonnet syndrome (Ricard 2009). Among those with more severe visual loss, this increases to approximately 50–60% of patients. CBS occurs mostly in people who have developed severe visual loss involving central vision in both eyes of which AMD is a cause (Ricard 2009). Table 3.5 (below) lists some of the features of CBS.

Table 3.5: Common features of Charles Bonnet syndrome

- Patients experience complex visual hallucinations.
- Hallucinations include patterns such as brickwork and grids; letters; people who are sometimes distorted or incomplete; animals; objects; and landscapes
- There is no sound associated with these hallucinations.
- The hallucinations are caused by impulses from the visual cortex in the absence of visual stimulation.
- Hallucinations may start occurring soon after the onset of visual loss, but they can sometimes appear up to ten years later.

(Adapted from Ricard 2009)

Visual hallucinations can provoke anxiety and be unsettling, and lack of information about the condition can lead to even greater distress in older patients (Ricard 2009). They may believe they have a mental illness, such as dementia, and that they are not only losing their sight, but also their mind (Ricard 2009). Recent research evidence suggests that among those suffering from CBS, 60% feared being labelled as insane if they admitted to having hallucinations, only 30% had ever revealed their condition to anyone else, and 30% lived in fear of impending insanity (Menon 2005).

There is currently no treatment for CBS. However, the nurse can still play a crucial role in alleviating the anxiety experienced by older patients by informing them about the condition and reassuring them about their mental state. The following reassuring statements may be offered:

- It is estimated that 50–60% of people suffering from severe visual loss will experience hallucinations.
- These visual hallucinations appear to abate after a while – for 60% of people they stop after 18 months.

- The visual hallucinations are purely a visual symptom and not due to any mental health problem.

- Some patients are able to find ways of controlling their hallucinations or of distinguishing between a real sight and a hallucination. 'Tricks' reported by sufferers include going into a brighter environment creating a distraction, looking directly at the images and making some form of eye movement. These suggestions may not work for all patients (Menon 2005, Ffytche 2008).

Such information should help to reduce the older patient's anxiety about their mental state. They will also feel better equipped to develop ways of managing their hallucinations and may become more confident in using their residual vision (Ricard 2009). At present, the condition remains largely unrecognised and further awareness of it should encourage patients to report their fears. The RCO and the Macular Disease Society have initiated a campaign to increase awareness of CBS among eye care staff (Ricard 2009).

Health education

The health and social care professional's role in providing health education is significant, since the aim is to restore sufficient independence to re-establish a reasonable quality of life (Watkinson 2010). Health education should also embrace family members, since the family are often the primary caregivers (Creuss et al. 2006). Wet AMD has a major impact on the lives of those with this disease, although this is largely underestimated by the public and clinicians (Creuss et al. 2006). Wet AMD patients have approximately one-third of the ability of people with normal vision to perform everyday activities, such as reading a newspaper, cooking, reading street signs, and walking down steps and kerbs in low light (Creuss et al. 2006). They have less than half the ability of people with normal vision to perform everyday 'distance' activities such as recognising faces, watching television, and taking part in outdoor activities (Creuss et al. 2006). Older patients therefore require more practical support and assistance in undertaking daily activities than those with normal vision.

Giving advice about overcoming such problems of daily living, especially reading and writing, and enhancing visual rehabilitation is paramount. Patients should be referred to the low vision hospital clinic, the visually impaired team, social services and the rehabilitation team. Advice can be provided on magnifying devices and large-print materials to assist with reading. Audiotaped books, newspapers and magazines are also available. Other appliances, such as liquid level indicators, talking watches, clocks, kitchen scales and microwave ovens, may help to compensate for the loss of detailed vision.

Putting patients in touch with support groups such as the AMD Alliance and the Royal National Institute of Blind People (RNIB) is advantageous. The Macular Disease Society (MDS) can offer essential help and support in meeting a wide range of needs, and setting up patient support groups in hospital eye units (Creuss et al. 2006). Advising older people to visit the optician every two years for an eye test is also important, particularly as eye tests are free for people over the age of 60 in the UK (RNIB 2008).

The public education role should not be underestimated in promoting early detection and treatment of AMD to avert the risk of visual loss. Opportunities to disseminate information at public healthcare seminars are invaluable. On average, it takes 14 to 15 months for those with untreated AMD to progress to legal blindness or worsened vision. Early detection through periodic eye examination is critical, as the patient with wet AMD can begin to lose vision in as little as three months after detection. Early intervention is the key to preserving vision.

Managing older patients undergoing intra-vitreal therapy
Assessment procedures
The following information should be documented:

- A full patient history
- Presenting ocular symptoms
- Ocular medication regime
- Other current medication
- Medical history
- Social history
- Family history of ocular problems
- Allergies.

Having documented this information, other procedures to be performed include:

- Recording visual acuity using LogMAR or Snellen chart. The Snellen chart is used to test central visual acuity. It consists of lines of letters or numbers, graded in size according to the distance at which they can be discriminated by a normal eye. The LogMAR is an algorithm for the logarithm of the minimum angle of resolution (MAR). The distance visual acuity of patients assessed using a LogMAR test is expressed as a logarithmic value. The smaller the letters on the chart and the further away they are, the smaller will be the angle presented to the eye by the letters on the chart, and thus the smaller the value of the LogMAR score associated with it.

- Measuring intra-ocular pressure (IOP) to check and monitor IOP in patients with existing glaucoma. If the IOP is elevated, appropriate treatment is administered.
- Checking for relative afferent pupillary defect to exclude the possibility of damage to the optic nerve.
- Dilating the pupil with tropicamide 1% and phenylephrine 2.5% eye drops to ensure a good view of the retina and to observe for the pulsating of the central retinal artery.
- Performing fluorescein dye angiography.
- Optical coherence tomography – this has to be undertaken by a specialist healthcare professional or technician.

Administering an intravitreal injection

The procedure is approached like a minor operation and a well-established care protocol is followed. The treatment room is cleaned, using the damp dusting technique, and equipment is assembled and aseptically prepared.

Medical staff will discuss the care plan with the patient. The healthcare professional is ideally placed to support the older patient psychologically and explain the risks and benefits of the course of treatment. All new patients will be taken through a step-by-step guide to the procedure. This approach enables understanding, supports self-management and patient education, and empowers the patient. Evidence-based information leaflets are provided, and advice is given about smoking cessation and eating a healthy diet. For older patients with a language barrier or learning disability, the individual's relatives, or a hospital interpreter, will be asked to attend and assist with the information-giving process. Informed consent is obtained before every intra-vitreal anti-VEGF therapy procedure, once a firm diagnosis has been established.

It is essential that patients are given time to comprehend the information on treatment modalities and the prognosis for maintenance of their sight. Patient identity is confirmed using a checklist against which the older patient's details are verified verbally, as per local policy.

Ocular preparation

Tropicamide 1% and phenylephrine 2.5% eye drops are instilled into the affected eye approximately 15 minutes before the procedure, to maximise pupillary dilation. Best practice also consists of instilling copious tetracaine hydrochloride 1% (a topical anaesthetic) eye drops over 5 to 10 minutes to minimise pain (RCO 2009). Studholme (2008) suggests that most patients remember the experience of pain when the needle is inserted. Maximum topical anaesthesia is therefore vital to optimise comfort during the procedure.

The appropriate eye is marked to ensure the correct patient receives treatment to the correct site. There is also a risk of infection following the intra-vitreal injection. Thus, patients are prescribed chloramphenicol 0.5% eye drops both before and after treatment.

The healthcare professional's presence throughout the procedure will help to ensure patient confidence, enhance safety, and maintain comfort and full co-operation. Sometimes, if needed, holding the patient's hand during this procedure can provide much reassurance. However, patient dignity and communication preferences must always be respected and prioritised.

Following the injection, the patient is monitored for 15 minutes for any adverse reactions, which are not commonly experienced. Occasionally, a patient may feel faint, and, very rarely, anaphylactic shock may occur.

Post-procedure advice

- Appropriate analgesia, such as paracetamol, may be required for feelings of grittiness in the eye, which last for approximately 24 hours.

- Focusing may be difficult for 3 to 4 hours afterwards until the pupil returns to normal.

- The patient should refrain from rubbing the treated eye because of the risk of corneal abrasion following topical anaesthesia.

- Small black or transparent dots may be noticed in the patient's visual field. These represent little drops of ranibizumab, or small air bubbles, in the vitreous humour.

- Generally, symptoms disappear within one to two days.

- Dark glasses should be worn in sunny weather to avoid direct ultra-violet rays.

- Provide an Amsler grid to self-monitor any deviation in vision.

- Contact telephone numbers should also be provided for use in the event of any deviation from the normal.

- In case of excruciating pain, sudden loss of vision or any further deterioration, the patient must attend the eye emergency department immediately, without an appointment.

- A quiet day following the procedure is advisable.

- Avoid swimming or splashing water into the eye for five days to prevent any infection.

- Patients are advised to attend all follow-up appointments and complete the course of treatment.

Future perspectives on AMD

While monthly injections of intra-vitreal anti-VEGF therapy for neovascular AMD have produced superior visual outcomes compared with previous therapies, the frequent clinic visits and injections required can place tremendous pressure on patients and the healthcare system.

Anti-VEGF agents are becoming cheaper and more widely available. However, an increasing number of older patients will need to rely on them, and the burden on the healthcare system will therefore increase. Furthermore, there are currently no approved treatments for geographic (dry) AMD although it may be possible to reduce the progression of dry AMD with a multivitamin integration, and many molecules are being tested (Querques et al. 2011).

Nevertheless, there will be a continuing demand for the healthcare system to provide appropriate services for older people with dry AMD, whose vision will continue to decline and reduce their quality of life over time. The advent of stem cell therapy offers some hope for the future treatment of AMD. However, for stem cell therapy to succeed in AMD patients with advanced degeneration, it is critical to develop a means of restoring the higher neuronal connections and pathways. This will clearly pose the biggest challenge to stem cell researchers for the future.

The primary challenge for all health and social care professionals is to take a collaborative approach to raising public awareness of the nature of AMD. This will facilitate prompt referral and diagnosis, and initiate prompt and appropriate treatment. Healthcare professionals are in an ideal position to recognise the symptoms and make immediate referrals for specialist care.

The macular nurse specialist, in particular, needs to engage in proactive strategic planning in order to maximise effective management of AMD clinics. Ongoing audit will be pivotal to ensuring the maintenance of standards and the delivery of high-quality care. Above all, showing compassion and empathy, and gaining insight into older patients' fears about going blind, will remain significant challenges for the future.

Conclusion

In summary, this chapter has focused on the clinical management of older people with dry and wet AMD. An overview of this condition was provided, covering its pathogenesis, classification, clinical features, aetiology and diagnosis.

Treatment of this ocular disease was discussed at some length, with reference to current and future perspectives, supported by a growing evidence base. The health and social care professional's role in the clinical management of older people with dry and wet

AMD was highlighted as significant and evolving. The provision of health education, effective communication, and counselling skills to help patients adjust to visual loss and its effect on quality of life all emerged as key elements. A more focused discussion of the care and management of older people undergoing intra-vitreal therapy was subsequently presented, with reference to the healthcare professional's role and specific skills required during this procedure.

In conclusion, it is important to reiterate that an undoubted increase in the incidence of AMD in older people will necessitate serious consideration of the future financial burden of visual impairment for the United Kingdom. Certainly the advent of Aflibercept as the latest anti-VEGF treatment for wet AMD, appears to represent a significant step towards making the treatment more cost-effective overall, as injections become two-monthly after the first three consecutive months of treatment.

As for stem cell therapy, research should defininitely continue in the form of small clinical trials. So far, the results of ongoing trials appear to be encouraging, and have certainly helped establish the safety of the procedure. However, the evidence seems to suggest that it is far too early to declare stem cell treatment as a viable cure for wet AMD.

Clearly, AMD is one of the major pathologies of retinal origin, accounting for most irreversible visual loss. The other major pathology is glaucoma, which will be discussed in the next chapter.

References

AMD.org (2010).
www.amd.org/living-with-amd/resources-and-tools/31-amsler-grid.html
(Last accessed 24 March 2014).

Berman, K. & Brodaty, H. (2006). Psychosocial effects of age-related macular degeneration. *International Psychogeriatrics.* **18** (3), 415–28.

Bosely, S. (2009). 'Antioxidants can slow the loss of sight in old age, scientists find.' *Guardian.* 19 June 2009.

Boyer, D.S., Heier, J.S., Brown, D.M., Francom, S.F., Lanchulev, T. & Rubio, R.G. (2009). A Phase IIIb study to evaluate the safety of ranibizumab in subjects with neovascular age-related macular degeneration. *Ophthalmology.* **116**, 1731–39.

Bressler, N.M. (2002). Early detection and treatment of neovascular age-related macular degeneration. *Journal of the American Board of Family Practice.* **15** (2), 142–52.

Brown, D.M., Michels, M., Kaiser, P.K., Heier, J.S. & Lanchulev, T. (2009). Ranibizumab versus verteporfin photodynamic therapy for neovascular age-related macular degeneration: Two-year results of the ANCHOR study. *Ophthalmology.* **116**, 57–65.

Bunce, C. & Wormald, R. (2008). Causes of blind certifications in England and Wales: April 1999–March 2000. *Eye.* **22** (7), 905–11.

CATT Research Group (2011). Ranibizumab and bevacizumab for neovascular age-related macular degeneration. *New England Journal of Medicine.* **364** (20), 1897–1908.

Chen, E., Brown, D.M. & Wong, T.P. (2010). Lucentis using Visudyne study: Determining the threshold-dose fluence of verteporfin photodynamic therapy combined with intra-vitreal ranibizumab for exudative macular degeneration. *Clinical Ophthalmology*. **4**, 1073–79.

Chong, E.W., Wong, T.Y., Kreis, A.J., Simpson, J.A. & Guymer, R.H. (2007). Dietary antioxidants and primary prevention of age related macular degeneration: systematic review and meta-analysis. *British Medical Journal*. **335** (7623), 755–62.

Chopdar, A., Chakravarthy, U. & Verma, D. (2003). Age-related macular degeneration. *British Medical Journal*. **326** (7387), 485–88.

Congdon, N., O'Colmain, B. & Klaver, C.C. (2004). Causes and prevalence of visual impairment among adults in the United States. *Archives of Ophthalmology*. **122** (4), 477–85.

Creuss, A., Xu, X. & Mones, J. (2006). Humanistic burden and health resource utilisation among neovascular age-related macular degeneration (AMD) patients: results from a multi-country cross-sectional study. *Association for Research in Vision and Ophthalmology Annual Meeting*: Abstract 2199. Fort Lauderdale, Florida FL, April 30–May 4 2006.

Ffytche, D. (2008). 'Charles Bonnet syndrome'. *Macular Degeneration Society Digest*. **6**, 27–32.

Hayman, K., Kerse, N. & Le Grow, S. (2007). Depression in older people: visual impairment and subjective ratings of health. *Optometry and Vision Science*. **84** (11), 1024–30.

Huang, L.L., Coleman, H.R. & Kim, J. (2008). Oral supplementation of lutein/zeaxanthin and omega-3 long chain polyunsaturated fatty acids in persons aged 60 years or older, with or without AMD. *Investigative Ophthalmology & Visual Science*. **49**, 3864–69.

Kanski, J. & Bowling, B. (2011). *Clinical Ophthalmology: A Systematic Approach*. 7th edn. London: Elsevier.

Khan, J.C., Shahid, H. & Thurlby, D.A. (2006). Age-related macular degeneration and sun exposure, iris colour, and skin sensitivity to sunlight. *British Journal of Ophthalmology*. **90** (1), 29–32.

Marsden, J. (2006). *Ophthalmic Care*. Chichester: Wiley.

Menon, G. (2005). Complex visual hallucinations in the visually impaired: a structured history-taking approach. *Archives of Ophthalmology*. **123** (3): 349–55.

Mitchell, J. & Bradley, C. (2006). Quality of life in age-related macular degeneration: a review of the literature. *Health and Quality of Life Outcomes*. **4**, 97.

Mooney, I. & LaMotte, L. (2011). Emerging options for the management of age-related macular degeneration with stem cells. *Stem Cells and Cloning: Advances and Applications*. **4**, 1–10.

National Institute for Health and Care Excellence (2008). Ranibizumab and Pegaptanib for the Treatment of Age-Related Macular Degeneration. Technology appraisal guidance 155. London: NICE.

National Institute for Health and Care Excellence (2013). Aflibercept solution for injection for treating wet age-related macular degeneration. NICE technology appraisal guidance 294. www.nice.org.uk/nicemedia/live/14227/64572/64572.pdf (Last accessed: 21 April 2014).

National Institutes of Health (2007). Study of fenretinide in the treatment of geographic atrophy associated with dry age-related macular degeneration. www.clinicaltrials.gov/ct2/show/NCT00429936?term=fenretinide&rank=10. (Last accessed: 21 April 2014).

Patel, S. (2009). Combination therapy for age-related macular degeneration. *Retina*. **29** (6), S45–48.

Querques, G., Avellis, F.O., Querques, L., Bandello, F. & Souied, E.H. (2011). Age-related macular degeneration. *Clinical Ophthalmology*. **5**, 593–601.

Radu, R.A., Han, Y. & Bui, T.V. (2005). Reductions in serum vitamin A arrest accumulation of toxic retinal fluorophores:

A potential therapy for treatment of lipofuscin-based retinal diseases. *Investigative Ophthalmology & Visual Science.* **46**, 4393–401.

Ricard, P. (2009). Vision loss and visual hallucinations: the Charles Bonnet Syndrome. *Community Eye Health.* **22** (69), 14.

Riordan-Eva, P. & Whitcher, J. (2008). *Vaughan and Asbury's General Ophthalmology.* 17th edn. New York, NY: Lange Medical Books/McGraw-Hill.

Rosenfeld, P.J., David, M. & Brown, D.M. (2006). Ranibizumab for neovascular age-related macular degeneration. *New England Journal of Medicine.* **355**, 1419–31.

Royal College of Ophthalmologists (2009). *Age-related macular degeneration: Guidelines for Management.* London: RCO.

Royal National Institute of Blind People (2008). 'Eye examinations'. http://www.rnib.org.uk/eyehealth/eyeexaminations/Pages/eye_examinations.aspx (Last accessed 25 March 2014).

Schmidt-Erfurth, U.M., Richard, G. & Augustin, A. (2007). Guidance for the treatment of neo-vascular macular degeneration. *Acta Ophthalmologica Scandinavica.* **85**, 486–94.

Singer, M. (2009). Horizon extension trial of ranibizumab (Lucentis) for neo-vascular age-related macular degeneration (AMD): Two-year safety and efficacy results. Investigative *Ophthalmology & Visual Science.* E-Abstract 3093.

Studholme, S. (2008). Comparison of methods of local anaesthesia used for cataract extraction. *Journal of Perioperative Practice.* **18** (1), 17–21.

Takeda, A.L., Colquitt, J., Clegg, A.J. & Jones, J. (2007). Pegaptanib and ranibizumab for neo-vascular age-related macular degeneration: A systematic review. *British Journal of Ophthalmology.* **91**, 1177–82.

Tanito, M., Li, F. & Anderson, R.E. (2010). Protection of retinal pigment epithelium by OT-551 and its metabolite TEMPOL-H against light-induced damage in rats. *Experimental Eye Research.* **91**, 111–14.

Watkinson, S. (2010). Management of older people with dry and wet age-related macular degeneration. *Nursing Older People.* **22** (5), 21–26.

Watkinson, S. & Scott, E. (2010). Care of patients undergoing intra-vitreal therapy. *Nursing Standard.* **24** (25), 42–47.

Wong, W.T., Kam, W. & Cunningham, D. (2010). Treatment of geographic atrophy by the topical administration of OT-551: Results of a Phase II clinical trial. *Investigative Ophthalmology & Visual Science.* **51**, 6131–39.

Chapter 4

Improving the care of older people with chronic open-angle glaucoma

Susan Watkinson

This chapter covers

- Introduction
- Overview of chronic open-angle glaucoma
- Pathophysiology
- Clinical features
- Risk factors
- Diagnosis
- Referral issues
- Clinical management of chronic open-angle glaucoma
- Approaches to treatment
- Effects on quality of life
- The health and social care professional's role
- Commitment to taking the prescribed treatment
- Support services for older people with glaucoma
- Future perspectives
- Conclusion

Introduction

In the previous chapter, age-related macular degeneration (AMD) was discussed at length – as a major pathology resulting in severe visual loss. After AMD, glaucoma is another principal reason for people having to register as blind. This chapter will focus on the care and clinical management of older people with chronic open-angle glaucoma (COAG). An overview of the condition, its pathogenesis, clinical features, aetiology and diagnosis will be provided. Current approaches to treatment will be outlined and future perspectives discussed. The health and social care professional's role in the clinical management of older people with this condition will then be considered.

Overall, patient education and promotion of adherence to medical therapy are paramount in establishing the confidence and independence required for the long-term self-management of COAG, as the majority of older people with this condition are based in the community.

Finally, some future perspectives on the role of the health and social care professional will be offered.

Overview of chronic open-angle glaucoma

Chronic open-angle glaucoma (COAG) is a common and potentially blinding condition. It is usually asymptomatic until it reaches an advanced stage, and many people will be unaware that there is a problem with their eyes until severe visual damage has occurred. Ocular hypertension (OHT) is a major risk factor for developing COAG, although COAG can occur with or without raised intra-ocular pressure (NICE 2009).

Approximately 10% of blindness registrations in the United Kingdom are attributed to glaucoma. Around 2% of people over the age of 40 have COAG, rising to almost 10% in people aged over 75 in white Europeans. The prevalence may be higher in people of black African or black Caribbean descent, or those with a family history of glaucoma. With changes in demographics, the number of individuals affected is expected to rise. Based on these estimates, 480,000 people are currently affected by COAG in England, and there are more than a million glaucoma-related hospital out-patient visits in the hospital eye service annually (NICE 2009).

People diagnosed with COAG require lifelong monitoring to detect the progression of visual damage. Once sight has been lost, it cannot be restored. It is therefore vital to control and prevent the condition, or at least keep ongoing damage to a minimum (NICE 2009).

Pathophysiology

COAG is a progressive disease in which a degenerative process takes place in the trabecular meshwork of the eye, with extracellular material being deposited in the meshwork and beneath the endothelial lining of Schlemm's canal. This leads to reduced aqueous drainage and a rise in intra-ocular pressure (IOP), with a gradual reduction in visual field (Riordan-Eva & Whitcher 2008).

The major mechanism of visual loss in glaucoma is retinal ganglion cell apoptosis, leading to thinning of the inner nuclear and nerve fibre layers of the retina and loss of axons in the optic nerve. The optic disc becomes atrophic, and the optic cup enlarges. In COAG, the IOP does not usually rise above 30mmHg, and retinal ganglion cell damage develops over a long period of time (Salmon 2008).

The drainage angle is formed by the iris and cornea (see Figure 4.1).

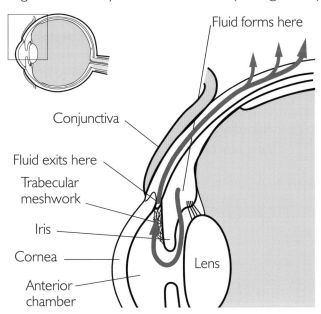

Figure 4.1: The drainage angle

The anterior chamber lies behind the cornea and in front of the iris. The posterior chamber lies between the iris, lens and ciliary body (James & Bron 2011). Aqueous humour is present in both chambers, and vitreous humour exists in the vitreous cavity. IOP is determined by the rate of aqueous production and the resistance to outflow of aqueous from the eye (Salmon 2008).

Formation and flow of aqueous

Aqueous is produced by the ciliary body. An ultrafiltrate of plasma is produced in the stroma of the ciliary processes and modified by the barrier function and secretory processes of the ciliary epithelium (Salmon 2008). The aqueous enters the posterior chamber and passes through the pupil into the anterior chamber and from there to the trabecular meshwork in the anterior chamber angle, which is where the iris meets the cornea.

The trabecular meshwork is made up of perforated sheets of collagen and elastic tissue, covered by trabecular cells, which form a filter with a decreasing pore size as the Schlemm's canal is approached (Salmon 2008). Contraction of the ciliary muscle through its insertion into the trabecular meshwork increases pore size in the meshwork and hence the rate of aqueous drainage. Passage of aqueous into Schlemm's canal depends on cyclic formation of transcellular channels in the endothelial lining. Efferent channels from Schlemm's canal (about 30 collector channels and 12 aqueous veins) conduct fluid directly into the venous system. Some aqueous passes between the bundles of the ciliary muscle into the suprachoroidal space and then into the venous system of the ciliary body, choroid, and sclera (uveoscleral flow).

The major resistance to aqueous outflow from the anterior chamber is the juxtacanalicular tissue adjacent to the endothelial lining of Schlemm's canal, rather than the venous system (Salmon 2008). However, the pressure in the episcleral venous system determines the minimum level of IOP that can be achieved by medical therapy (Salmon 2008).

Clinical features

Clinical features include:

- Onset in adulthood
- Slight to moderate increase in IOP (24–32mmHg)
- Open drainage angle
- Loss of visual field
- Cupping of the optic disc and loss of peripheral vision.

(Kanski & Bowling 2011)

However, between one-third and half of patients with glaucoma have IOP of less than 21mmHg.

Risk factors

Ocular hypertension (OHT) is a major risk factor for developing COAG. Ocular hypertension is elevated eye pressure in the absence of visual field loss or glaucomatous optic nerve damage. It is estimated that between 3 and 5% of those over the age of 40 have OHT, around one million people in England (NICE, 2009). This represents a major risk for the future development of COAG.

Classic risk factors include:

- Being aged over 60
- Being African or African-Caribbean
- Being of Hispanic ethnicity

- Having a family history of glaucoma
- Increased cup-disc ratio (the diameter of the cupped portion of the disc compared with its overall diameter)
- Having thin central corneal thickness, which leads to underestimation of IOP
- Black patients in particular may have thinner average central corneal thickness, resulting in under-diagnosis of elevated pressure.

(Adapted from Kanski & Bowling 2011)

Contributory risk factors include:

- Systemic hypertension
- Cardiovascular disease
- Diabetes
- Myopia
- Smoking
- Long-term corticosteroid use.

Diagnosis

Diagnosis cannot be based on increased IOP alone. Two or more of the following investigations will be performed to determine the diagnosis for older people with OHT, suspected COAG, or COAG.

- IOP measurement using Goldmann applanation tonometry
- Peripheral anterior chamber configuration and depth assessments using gonioscopy
- Visual field measurement using standard automated perimetry
- Optic nerve assessment, with dilatation, using stereoscopic slit-lamp biomicroscopy with fundus examination
- Obtaining of an optic nerve head image.

A positive diagnosis is usually made when two of the following signs are present: elevated IOP, degeneration of the optic disc and visual field loss. Importantly, when abnormal features are identified at the optic disc, a judgement has to be made as to whether the abnormalities are likely to represent progression of the condition (Riordan-Eva & Whitcher 2008). Figures 4.2 and 4.3 (page 70) show a normal optic disc compared with a cupped glaucomatous disc.

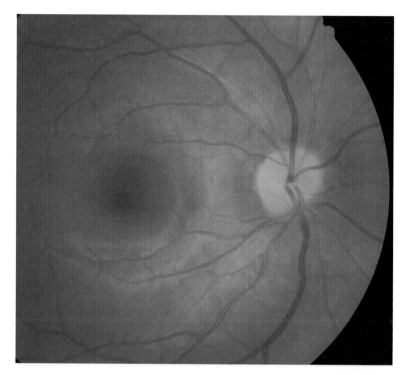

Figure 4.2: A normal optic disc

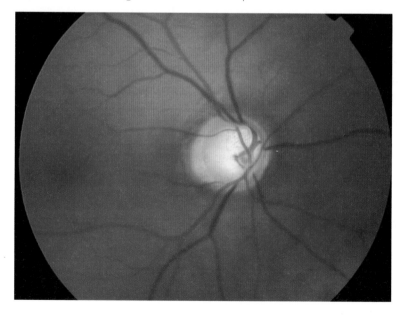

Figure 4.3: A cupped, glaucomatous disc

Referral issues

In the UK, the vast majority of older people with suspected glaucoma will be identified by community optometrists during a routine eye examination (Parkins & Edgar 2011). They are then normally referred to the Hospital Eye Service (HES) for formal diagnosis and ongoing management. Currently, as a national screening scheme for glaucoma appears not to be cost-effective, many older people with suspected glaucoma will be identified via a process of opportunistic case-finding (Parkins & Edgar 2011).

The College of Optometrists recommends that good practice should include tonometry to measure the IOP, assessment of the central visual field using perimetry with threshold control and assessment of the optic nerve head. However, apart from the latter, the optometrist is not obliged to carry out the remaining specific tests during an NHS or private eye examination. More significantly, non-contact tonometry (NCT) is most commonly used by UK optometrists in community practice, whilst contact tonometry is used in hospital clinics for measuring the IOP (Willis et al. 2000). Contact tonometry is considered the most accurate method, with the Goldmann Applanation Tonometry (GAT) technique regarded as the 'gold standard'. Consequently, there have been some problems with reliance on single test result for tonometry or visual field assessment (Parkins & Edgar 2011).

Published research suggests there is a need for improvement in the quality of glaucoma-related referrals from primary care optometry, but often it is only by repeating measurements that the quality of referrals can be improved (Ang et al. 2009). The two main issues affecting the quality of glaucoma-related referrals in England are contractual: firstly, there is the current lack of funding for repeat measurements; and, secondly, most optometry practices have chosen to use NCT, because it can often be delegated to non-qualified staff, which saves the optometrist's time (Myint et al. 2010).

Clinical management of COAG

The aim of treatment

The overall aim of treatment is to reduce the IOP sufficiently to achieve the 'target IOP range'. The target IOP is a dynamic, clinical judgment about what level of IOP is considered by the healthcare professional treating an individual to be sufficiently low to minimise or arrest disease progression or onset and avoid disability from sight loss within an individual's lifetime (NICE 2009). It may also be defined as the IOP at which the sum of the health-related quality of life (HRQOL) from preserved vision and the HRQOL from not having side-effects from treatment is maximised (Parikh et al. 2008). Randomised controlled trials provide good evidence to suggest that lowering IOP to target levels slows optic nerve and/or visual field damage. IOP also appears to be the only risk factor that can be easily modified and objectively monitored by eye care professionals, thereby minimising conversion rates of ocular hypertension (OHT) to glaucoma and disease progression in established glaucoma (Nemesure et al. 2007).

Target IOP has to be individualised, based on the patient's clinical profile. This can be formally calculated, using tables, graphs, or formulae. However, common practice is to reduce the IOP by at least 20% in mild, 30% in moderate, and more than 40% in severe glaucoma. Generally, the formulae and other methods will provide similar values (Parikh et al. 2008).

The higher the IOP, the larger the reduction required. For example, if the patient has an IOP of 40mmHg initially, a larger percentage reduction would be required. In this case, a 20% reduction from 40mmHg would only bring the IOP into the 30mmHg range, which is not adequate.

Where advanced glaucoma is evident in a young or middle-aged patient, the IOP may need to be reduced by 50% from the baseline. However, the existence of the same clinical findings in a very old patient may necessitate setting the target to an even higher level to ensure minimal hampering of the quality of life for that individual (Parikh et al. 2008).

Approaches to treatment

Intra-ocular pressure can be lowered by decreasing the production of aqueous humour, increasing its outflow, or both. Approaches to treatment include:

- Ocular hypotensive treatment
- Laser surgery
- Incisional surgery
- A combination of the above three.

(Sharts-Hopko & Glynn-Milley 2009).

Ocular hypotensive treatment

Adherence to this approach to treatment is vital. Topical prostaglandin analogues such as latanoprost 0.005% eye drops are usually prescribed initially because of their low incidence of side-effects and convenient once-daily instillation. These drugs increase the uveoscleral outflow of aqueous humour through the ciliary muscle by relaxing the muscle or remodelling the surrounding extracellular matrix (Sharts-Hopko & Glynn-Milley 2009).

Topical beta-adrenergic antagonists, such as timolol hemihydrate, are also often used initially. They lower the production of aqueous humour by blocking beta receptors in the ciliary epithelium and mediating sympathetic nerve stimulation.

Carbonic anhydrase inhibitors lessen aqueous humour production by interfering with an enzyme (carbonic anhydrase) that is involved in sodium and fluid transport in the ciliary body. Topical dorzolamide 2% eye drops are generally used as adjunct therapy with other drugs to lower the IOP (Sharts-Hopko & Glynn-Milley 2009). This involves making a clinical decision about what level of IOP is considered to be low by the healthcare professional treating the person.

The aim is to minimise or arrest disease progression or onset and avoid disability from sight loss within a person's expected lifetime (NICE 2009).

Laser surgery

This is indicated when COAG is unresponsive to drug therapy, when patients are unable to tolerate the drugs, or because of non-adherence to the prescribed regimen. Specifically, argon laser trabeculoplasty is performed to cut several tiny holes in the trabecular meshwork. This causes scars, which, on contraction, will widen the channels of the meshwork and make it easier for the aqueous humour to flow out and reduce the IOP (Kanski & Bowling 2011). Usually, one eye is treated at a time to allow the procedure's effect to be assessed and to avoid total visual impairment. Results are evaluated after six weeks.

Incisional surgery

This is filtering surgery (trabecular meshwork or Schlemm's canal surgery, trabeculectomy, and implantation of shunts) aimed at draining aqueous humour from the eye. It is usually considered when drug therapy and laser surgery have failed. Performing a trabeculectomy is the most common treatment. This involves excising a tiny portion of the trabecular meshwork to create an opening and provide an alternative route for the drainage of aqueous humour. This reduces the pressure and prevents further damage. The aim is to achieve incomplete healing of the surgical wound, with the formation of a bleb at the excision site. Gonioscopy should also be performed annually because the anterior chamber becomes shallow with age (Kanski & Bowling 2011).

Treatment and quality of life issues

Overall, achieving target IOP range involves establishing a fine balance between prescribing appropriate medication and using the other treatment approaches just described to lower the IOP whilst preserving patients' vision and ensuring an acceptable quality of life. However, patients' expectations of treatment are sometimes at variance with the goals of healthcare professionals. In Bhargava et al.'s study (2006), 82 patients were questioned about their biggest anxiety related to therapy. The significant finding was that most patients were concerned about the onset of immediate visual impairment impacting their freedom and the risk of blindness.

Clearly, quality of life issues also emerge from long-term therapy. Aspinall *et al.* (2008) categorised patients into two groups based on their main priorities, which were 'reading and seeing detail', and 'outdoor mobility'. As the second group of patients lost more of their peripheral vision, their priority changed from 'outdoor mobility' to 'reading and seeing detail'. These patients gradually became more willing to comply with prescribed glaucoma therapy in order to avoid going blind and preserve reasonable visual quality of life in the longer term. In other words, they were prepared to sacrifice their outdoor interests, pursuits and occupations for the sake of preserving their ability to read and see detail (Aspinall *et al.* 2008).

Monitoring

Although not all older people with COAG or suspected OHT are recommended to receive medication (NICE 2009), assessment of the IOP, optic disc and visual field is necessary at the following intervals:

- Between 12 and 24 months if there is a low risk of conversion to COAG
- Between 6 and 12 months if there is a high risk of conversion to COAG.

If no change in the parameters has been detected after three to five years (or before, if confirmed normal), the person should be discharged from active glaucoma care to community optometric care (NICE 2009). At discharge, people not recommended for treatment, and whose condition is considered stable, are advised to visit the primary care optometrist annually to check for any changes in their condition (NICE 2009).

Effects on quality of life

The shock of being diagnosed with glaucoma and the fear of going blind can have an adverse effect. Depression is common in older people with visual impairment (Hayman *et al.* 2007) and can profoundly affect their quality of life, general and visual functioning, and the ability to benefit from a range of rehabilitative processes (Evans *et al.* 2007).

In highlighting this problem, Evans *et al.* (2007) reported that 13.5% of visually impaired older people had a score of 6 or more on the Geriatric Depression Scale, compared with 4.6% of those with good vision, and that this was particularly linked to problems experienced with daily functioning. Activities such as driving or playing certain sports may become more challenging. Loss of contrast sensitivity, problems with glare and light sensitivity may also affect daily functioning. If older people have problems with night-time vision, it may be better to consider doing most of their travelling during the daytime. Sunglasses or tinted lenses can help with glare and contrast.

The health and social care professional's role

Patient education

The health and social care professional should promote eye health by educating patients. Long-term management of this condition is paramount, since the majority of older people with COAG are in the community (Watkinson 2010). Offering older people and their relatives the opportunity to discuss the diagnosis, prognosis, available treatments and their associated side-effects, and providing them with relevant information at the initial and subsequent clinic visits, increases adherence to prescribed treatment (Watkinson 2010). The need for regular monitoring of the condition, as previously highlighted, should also be reinforced. Glaucoma can run in families, and family members may wish to be tested for the disease.

Information about side-effects of therapy

Useful information about the side-effects of therapy can be provided by the health and social care professional. For example, prostaglandin analogues, such as latanoprost, cause benign but irreversible darkening of the iris and increased growth and thickening of the eyelashes (Sharts-Hopko & Glynn-Milley 2009). Burning, stinging, and a foreign body sensation may also be inhibitors, and dorzolamide often gives rise to ocular burning and discomfort and altered taste. Carbonic anhydrase inhibitors are also contraindicated in people who are allergic to sulphur drugs (Sharts-Hopko & Glynn-Milley 2009). They may increase corneal oedema in low endothelial cell count and/or corneal endothelial dysfunction, as in Fuchs' dystrophy (Kulkarni et al. 2008).

Beta blocking drugs have few adverse ocular side-effects, but may have adverse systemic effects such as bradycardia, hypotension, bronchospasm and depression. They can also mask hypoglycaemia in insulin-dependent diabetes mellitus (Kulkarni et al. 2008). Since respiratory failure is also possible, these drugs are contraindicated in older people with asthma, chronic obstructive pulmonary disease, sinus bradycardia and heart block (Sharts-Hopko & Glynn-Milley 2009).

After laser trabeculoplasty, inflammation and soreness might be experienced, but these symptoms can be managed with non-steroidal anti-inflammatory drugs. Possible complications of a trabeculectomy include corneal damage, delayed healing, scarring and excess fluid loss from the eye (Sharts-Hopko & Glynn-Milley 2009).

Overcoming the barriers to adherence

The health and social care professional can help older patients to overcome barriers to adherence by providing them with the necessary information and support to develop good drop instillation techniques, thereby reducing anxiety and promoting self-confidence and longer-term independence. Teaching older people and relatives how to instil eye drops correctly, safely and at the appropriate time is essential for the treatment and control of COAG (Watkinson 2010).

Evidence suggests that compliance is enhanced when patients self-medicate (Friedman et al. 2008). Particularly in situations where an older person's physical or mental disability may compromise their ability to self-medicate, the support of committed family members or friends in drop instillation becomes even more critical. For example, liaising with relatives about continuity of care after surgery is advantageous because of the valuable contribution they can make in optimising the older person's adherence to prescribed treatment.

Observing the eyes daily for any signs of excessive swelling or stickiness, indicating infection, is important and may necessitate appropriate referral to the primary care physician. Relatives can also make an important contribution when the older person is hospitalised for treatment of a co-existing condition. The drug therapy prescribed for COAG may consist of several types of eye drops, which must continue to be administered throughout the hospital stay. Here, relatives can help with monitoring medication administration, thus ensuring the older person's adherence to ongoing management of the ocular condition.

Other key strategies for enhancing compliance and concordance are provision of written instructions about the treatment regimen and an easy medication schedule and reminder in the form of a hand-out (Kulkarni et al. 2008). The maintenance of a medication diary is particularly useful for a highly motivated patient. Kulkarni et al. (2008) also cite the use of medication monitors, alarm clocks and travel alert devices for patients who need reminders for therapy when travelling.

Developing a therapeutic relationship

Clearly, the prospect of losing one's sight is daunting and developing a therapeutic relationship with the older patient is therefore invaluable. The health and social care professional should strive to gain insight into the older person's feelings and their fears of blindness. Counselling skills, active listening and positive responses are pivotal (Watkinson 2010). Older people are usually better able to cope with their emotions when time is provided to allay their apprehensions and fears.

It is necessary to explore expectations of better vision associated with treatment in order to dispel false hopes that either medical or surgical intervention will improve existing vision (Watkinson & Scott 2010). Once sight has been lost, it cannot be recovered. However, it is equally important to stress that most patients treated for COAG will not go blind (NICE 2009). Thus, providing older people with opportunities to discuss any problems or concerns will enable the health and social care professional to offer advice and arrange for appropriate help and support.

Ongoing assessment

Targeted questions about the older person's vision and visual problems, especially at night and when walking down steps and pavement kerbs, are essential as part of ongoing assessment and evaluation of the condition. It is vital to explain the need to attend regular clinic appointments for assessment and further monitoring in order to identify any deterioration and potential threat to future sight-related quality of life. Older people with impaired vision are at an increased risk of falls, which can result in a decline in health status, daily functioning, lifestyle and quality of life (Roe et al. 2009).

Commitment to taking the prescribed treatment

Successful management of COAG depends very much on the older person's ability to commit to the treatment plan and prescribed medication regime. Commitment involves a combination of 'compliance', 'adherence' and 'concordance', three terms that are currently generating much debate amongst healthcare and social care professionals. Medication compliance concerns the accuracy with which a patient follows the treatment plan, while adherence is the extent to which the patient can continue the treatment (Kulkarni et al. 2008). The NHS prefers to use the term concordance when discussing patient involvement in the treatment process and participation with the healthcare professional in treatment decisions. The patient is also viewed as being partially responsible for monitoring and reporting back to the team (Kulkarni et al. 2008).

Regardless of the fine distinctions between these different terms, establishing a therapeutic relationship with the older person and utilising effective interpersonal skills for quality interaction are instrumental in achieving a successful patient–provider partnership (Seewoodhary & Watkinson 2011).

Poor adherence to therapy is a significant issue, particularly in patients with COAG (Gray et al. 2009), and it is very common (Olthoff et al. 2009). Treatment failure may necessitate unwarranted changes of medications, increased healthcare expenditure and risk to the patient if surgical intervention is required (Gray et al. 2009). Kulkarni et al. (2008) reported psychological, socioeconomic, poor health literacy, inadequate information and inadequate patient–provider relationships as factors preventing patients from accessing complete treatment.

Tsai et al. (2003) reported that patient compliance was affected by four types of barrier, in the following proportions: 49% due to social/environmental factors (lack of support, major life events and travel); 32% by regimen factors (complexity, costs and change in medication); 16% by individual patient factors (knowledge, memory, motivation); and 3% by medical provider factors (dissatisfaction, communication). A qualitative study by Lacey *et al.* (2009) identified many obstacles to adherence, including poor education, lack of motivation, forgetfulness and drop application.

Evidence also suggests that older people require more information on the correct administration of eye drops because difficulties are encountered when using the medication – for example, holding the bottle above the eye when applying the drops (Olthoff *et al.* 2009), 'drops falling on the cheek' and 'too many drops coming out' during instillation (Sleath *et al.* 2009). Simplification of dosing regimens, the use of reminder devices, education and individual care planning have all been found to contribute to some improvements in adherence rates (Gray *et al.* 2009).

Djafari *et al.* (2009) also found that patients using prostaglandin analogues or beta blockers adhered more to therapy than those using carbonic anhydrase inhibitors. Importantly, identification of specific obstacles to adherence early after diagnosis, and a tailored approach to patient care (with initial education about the consequences of non-adherence and longer-term feedback about drop efficacy), may improve patients' motivation for adherence (Lacey *et al.* 2009).

Support services for older people with glaucoma
The role of the Eye Clinic Liaison Officer

Eye Clinic Liaison Officers (ECLOs) can provide information on the impact of the eye condition and subsequent support for patients and their carers when sight loss first becomes a concern (Boyce 2011). Other ways of helping patients include assistance with completing documentation for Certificate of Vision Impairment (CVI) registration. This is invaluable and results in more expedient referral of blind and partially sighted older people to statutory and voluntary services. ECLOs can also give advice on reducing frequency of falls, emotional support, and guidance on accessing local and national support services (Boyce 2011).

Referral for social care support is important. If an older person with glaucoma experiences difficulty with performing daily tasks due to sight loss, the local authority low vision team should be contacted. Helpful advice and practical support can be given to help the person make the most of their existing vision. Information can also be provided about the financial help the older person may be eligible to receive, such as the Blind Person's Allowance.

Providing practical and emotional support to older people with sight loss due to glaucoma is beneficial in several ways. It increases their confidence and ability to self-manage their glaucoma, improves health outcomes, and promotes more independent living. Overall, the role of the ECLO is therefore instrumental in empowering older patients to establish and maintain sight-related quality of life.

Voluntary services

Informal care and support networks are also important. Charitable organisations, such as the Royal National Institute of Blind People (RNIB), the International Glaucoma Association (IGA) and local patient support groups, can provide additional help and support to improve the older person's quality of life. The IGA offers a patient helpline (called Sightline), runs awareness campaigns, holds IGA patient meetings, provides help with setting up support groups, supplies a wide range of patient literature, provides support for professional meetings, and equips eye units with an educational tool (compliance briefcase).

The Glaucoma Research Foundation (GRF) will also provide information for newly diagnosed glaucoma patients and send free educational booklets to the patient and a relative. Since there is an increased familial risk of developing COAG, relatives are advised to undergo regular sight tests every two to three years. Eye tests are free for first-degree relatives of people with glaucoma aged 40 years and over in England (NHS Choices 2008). If driving is essential for the older person, safety to drive should be verified by an ophthalmologist and the Driver and Vehicle Licensing Agency (2009) guidelines should be followed.

Health literacy

One of the major problems for older people with glaucoma is lack of health literacy. The impact of low health literacy on healthcare and outcomes is a cause for concern that spans all racial and ethnic groups. The National Eye Institute has found that poor health literacy is common among racial and ethnic minorities, older people and patients with chronic conditions such as diabetes (NEI 2006). This lack of health literacy is a barrier to accessing and receiving healthcare services and has been recognised as a problem impacting on healthcare quality and costs (NEI 2006).

Healthcare messages targeting older people should be culturally sensitive to the unique issues they face, such as anxiety about the loss of independence, unwillingness to seek medical help, and fear of the medical and healthcare system. There appears to be a fear of blindness among older people, and limited knowledge regarding age-related vision loss.

Lay knowledge and subjective assessment of risk have been identified as important motivators in influencing older people's healthcare decisions (NEI 2006). Public awareness and knowledge of glaucoma therefore remain a major concern both for ophthalmic healthcare professionals and other related health and social care professionals (Baker *et al.* 2010). More informed public health education programmes are required specifically to target issues relating to older people with glaucoma. This may be the only way to ensure effective delivery of community eye health information in the future.

Future perspectives

Raising public awareness through health promotion is a key consideration in order to reduce the socio-economic burden of this condition for the future. As COAG is a cause of irreversible optic nerve damage and progressive sight loss (Seewoodhary & Watkinson 2011), it represents a substantial potential cost for the healthcare service.

Although Baker *et al.* (2010) found greater public awareness of glaucoma, compared with findings from a previous study (Baker & Murdoch 2004), they still identified poor knowledge of the condition within lower social classes. Baker & Murdoch (2004) argue that, for any health promotion strategy to be successful, it needs to be supported by extensive public relations and promotional efforts, including media advocacy. Clearly, ophthalmic nurses and related health and social care professionals can make a significant, albeit challenging, contribution to public education (RCN 2009). Some of their main responsibilities will include provision of education through effective communication and interpersonal skills, and the promotion of health through exploration of health beliefs and attitudes.

In the UK, in particular, as previously discussed, the recently introduced Eye Clinic Liaison Officer can play a vital role in providing information for older people about their eye condition.

Reducing the socio-economic burden

Reducing the socio-economic burden of visual impairment due to COAG will be a key target to address for the future. This will mean understanding and overcoming the barriers to effective treatment in order to ensure optimal utilisation of finite human and financial resources for patients, practitioners and the healthcare system. Thus, some of the chief objectives must be:

● Utilising evidence-based guidelines for treating COAG to the full.

● Keeping the treatment plan straightforward and tailored to the patient's needs and preferences. For example, for patients with memory problems (such as Alzheimer's disease), prescribing fewer drops may mean better compliance.

● Recognising any potential obstacles to compliance and concordance at an early stage, and planning appropriate interventions to address these problems. For example, poor health literacy can be helped by organising patient education sessions.

- Monitoring the progress of the disease, maintaining quality of life, and initiating timely interventions as required. These measures are all instrumental in reducing the longer-term socio-economic burden of glaucoma.

(Adapted from Kulkarni et al. 2008)

Conclusion

In summary, this chapter has addressed the clinical management of older people with COAG. An overview of this condition was provided, with reference to the underlying pathophysiological changes taking place and the resulting significant clinical features. Risk factors, current methods of diagnosis, the existing debatable issues around glaucoma referral, and the importance of ongoing monitoring of the condition, were addressed. Approaches to treatment were then discussed, with reference to some of the main side-effects and limitations of the ocular drug therapy currently being prescribed. Key aspects of the health and social care professional's role in improving the care of older people with this condition were then explored.

In conclusion, it is important to reiterate that the role of the health and social care professional in the care and management of older people with COAG will become significantly more challenging in the future.

Early diagnosis and prompt treatment are vital to the preservation of sight in the longer term. Key elements in the provision of care are good communication, effective counselling skills, patient education and collaboration with other healthcare professionals to raise public awareness of the condition, and ongoing practical help and support to promote adherence to prescribed medical therapy. The primary aim is to empower older people to give them independence and long-term control over the self-management of their ocular condition.

The importance of achieving long-term control, and maintaining a sight-related quality of life, should not be underestimated when considering visual impairment due to ocular disease. This is equally true of the older person with diabetic retinopathy, where rigorous self-management of both the diabetes mellitus and resulting ocular pathology is crucial to maintaining a sight-related quality of life and reducing the risk of systemic complications. Managing the older person with diabetic retinopathy will be the focus of discussion in the next chapter.

References

Ang, G.S., Ng, W.S. & Azuara-Blanco, A. (2009). The influence of the new general ophthalmic services (GOS) contract in optometrist referrals for glaucoma in Scotland. *Eye*. **23**, 351–355.

Aspinall, P.A., Johnson, Z.K. & Azuara-Blanco, A. (2008). Evaluation of quality of life and priorities of patients with glaucoma. *Investigative Ophthalmology & Visual Science*. **49**, 1907–15.

Baker, H. & Murdoch, I.E. (2004). Can a public health package on glaucoma reach its target population? *Eye*. **18**, 478–82.

Baker, H., Cousens, S.N. & Murdoch, I.E. (2010). Poor public health knowledge about glaucoma; fact or fiction? *Eye*. **24**, 653–57.

Bhargava, J.S., Patel, B. & Foss, A.J. (2006). Views of glaucoma patients on aspects of their treatment: an assessment of patient preference by conjoint analysis. *Investigative Ophthalmology & Visual Science*. **47**, 2885–88.

Boyce, T. (2011). *Innovation and quality in sight loss and blindness services: Eye Clinic Liaison Officers*. London: RNIB.

Djafari, F., Lesk, M. & Harasymowycz, P. (2009). Determinants of adherence to glaucoma medical therapy in a long-term patient population. *Journal of Glaucoma*. **18** (3), 238–43.

Driver and Vehicle Licensing Agency (2009). At a Glance Guide to the Current Medical Standards of Fitness to Drive. www..gov.uk (Last accessed: 22 April 2014, search for 'fitness to drive').

Evans, J., Fletcher, A. & Wormald, R. (2007). Depression and anxiety in visually impaired older people. *Ophthalmology*. **114** (2), 283–88.

Friedman, D.S., Hahn, S.R. & Gelb, L. (2008). Doctor-patient communication, health-related beliefs, and adherence in glaucoma results from the Glaucoma Adherence and Persistency Study. *Ophthalmology*. **115**, 1320–27.

Gray, T., Orton, L. & Henson, D. (2009). Interventions for improving adherence to ocular hypotensive therapy. (Cochrane Review). The Cochrane Library. Issue 2 Chichester: John Wiley and Sons.

Hayman, K., Kerse, N. & LaGrow, S. (2007). Depression in older people: visual impairment and subjective ratings of health. *Optometry and Vision Science*. **84** (11), 1024–30.

International Glaucoma Association: The Charity For People With Glaucoma. www.glaucoma-association.com (Last accessed: 22 April 2014).

James, B. & Bron, A. (2011). *Lecture Notes on Ophthalmology*. 11th edn. Oxford: Wiley-Blackwell.

Kanski, J. & Bowling, B. (2011). *Clinical Ophthalmology: A Systematic Approach*. 7th edn. London: Elsevier.

Kulkarni, S.V., Damjii, K.F. & Buys, Y.M. (2008). Medical management of primary open-angle glaucoma: Best practices associated with enhanced patient compliance and persistency. *Patient Preference and Adherence*. **2**, 303–13.

Lacey, J., Cate, H. & Broadway, D. (2009). Barriers to adherence with glaucoma medications: a qualitative research study. *Eye*. **23** (4), 924–32.

Myint, J., Edgar, D.F. & Kotecha, A. (2010). Barriers perceived by UK-based community optometrists to the detection of primary open-angle glaucoma. *Ophthalmic and Physiological Optics*. **30**, 847–53.

NHS Choices (2008): 'Am I Entitled to a Free NHS Sight Test? www.nhs.uk/chq/Pages/895.aspx?CategoryID=68&Sub CategoryID=157 (Last accessed: 14 April 2012).

National Eye Institute (2006). 'Effective Education to Target Populations: National Eye Health Education Program Five-Year Agenda 2006–2011'. NEI. www.nei.nih.gov/nehep/research/Effective_Education_to_Target_Populations.pdf (Last accessed: 22 April 2014).

Nemesure, B., Honkanen, R. & Hennis, A. (2007). Barbados Eye Studies Group Incident open-angle glaucoma and intra-ocular pressure. *Ophthalmology*. **114**, 1810–15.

National Institute for Health and Clinical Excellence (2009). *Glaucoma: Diagnosis and Management of Chronic Open-angle glaucoma and Ocular Hypertension. Clinical Guideline 85.* London: NICE.

Olthoff, C., Hoevenaars, J. & van den Borne, B. (2009). Prevalence and determinants of non-adherence to topical hypotensive treatment in Dutch glaucoma patients. *Graefe's Archive for Clinical and Experimental Ophthalmology.* **247** (2), 235–43.

Parikh, R.S., Parikh, S.R. & Navin, S. (May–June 2008). Practical approach to medical management of glaucoma. *Indian Journal of Ophthalmology.* **56** (3), 223–30.

Parkins, D.J. & Edgar, D.F. (2011). Comparison of the effectiveness of two enhanced glaucoma referral schemes. *Ophthalmic & Physiological Optics.* **31**, 343–52.

Riordan-Eva, P. & Whitcher, J. (2008). *Vaughan and Asbury's General Ophthalmology.* 17th edn. New York, NY: Lange Medical Books/McGraw-Hill.

Roe, B., Howell, F. & Riniotis, K. (2009). Older people and falls: health status, quality of life, lifestyle, care networks, prevention and views on service use following a recent fall. *Journal of Clinical Nursing.* **18** (16), 2261–72.

Royal College of Nursing (2009). 'The nature, scope and value of ophthalmic nursing'. London: RCN. www.rcn.org.uk/__data/assets/pdf_file/0010/258490/003521.pdf
(Last accessed 27 March 2014).

Salmon, J.F. (2008). 'Chapter 11 Glaucoma' in Riordan-Eva, P. & Whitcher, J. (2008). *Vaughan and Asbury's General Ophthalmology.* 17th edn. New York, NY: Lange Medical Books/McGraw-Hill, 212–28.

Seewoodhary, R. & Watkinson, S. (2011). Public health knowledge of glaucoma: implications for the ophthalmic nurse. *International Journal of Ophthalmic Practice.* **2** (4), 170–77.

Sharts-Hopko, N. & Glynn-Milley, C. (2009). Primary open-angle glaucoma. *American Journal of Nursing.* **109** (2), 40–47.

Sleath, B., Ballinger, R. & Covert, D. (2009). Self-reported prevalence and factors associated with nonadherence with glaucoma medications in veteran outpatients. *American Journal of Geriatric Pharmacotherapy.* **7** (2), 67–73.

Tsai, J.C., McClure, C.A. & Ramos, S.E. (2003). Compliance barriers in glaucoma: a systematic classification. *Journal of Glaucoma.* 12, 393–98.

Watkinson, S. (2010). Improving care of chronic open-angle glaucoma. *Nursing Older People.* **22** (8), 18–23.

Watkinson, S. & Scott, E. (2010). Care of patients undergoing intra-vitreal therapy. *Nursing Standard.* **24** (25), 42–47.

Willis, C.E. Rankin, S.J. & Jackson, A.J. (2000). Glaucoma in optometric practice: a survey of optometrists. *Ophthalmic & Physiological Optics.* **20**, 70–75.

Chapter 5

Older people with diabetic retinopathy

Susan Watkinson

This chapter covers

- Introduction
- Diabetes mellitus – an overview
- Diabetic retinopathy
- Retinal screening
- Clinical management and the role of the health and social care professional
- Health beliefs and attitudes
- Future perspectives
- Conclusion

Introduction

This chapter will focus on the management of older people with diabetic retinopathy. Initially, an overview of diabetes mellitus will be presented, including its epidemiology, main types, risk factors, blood glucose regulation, and complications. Diabetic retinopathy, as a major ocular complication of diabetes, will subsequently be addressed, with reference to its pathogenesis, risk factors and classification. This will be followed by a detailed discussion of the role of the health and social care professional in the clinical management of older people with diabetic retinopathy. Health education and effective communication and counselling skills are of central importance in helping older people gain control over the self-management of their diabetes in order to preserve vision and maintain quality of life for as long as possible.

Retinal screening, as a further significant aspect of health education, will also be discussed as a vital means of monitoring the development of diabetic retinopathy and its effects on vision, with a view to arranging clinical intervention to prevent further visual deterioration.

The chapter will conclude by examining future perspectives for older people with diabetic retinopathy.

Diabetes mellitus – an overview

Epidemiology

The estimated prevalence of diabetes mellitus worldwide for 2011 was 366 million and it is expected to affect 552 million people by 2030 (NICE 2008). In the UK it is estimated that one in 20 people has diabetes (Diabetes UK 2012). There are currently 3.2 million people diagnosed with diabetes in the UK and an estimated 630,000 people who have the condition, but do not know it (Diabetes UK 2014).

By 2025, it is estimated that the number of people with diabetes will have increased to 5 million (QOF 2011). Most of these cases will be type 2 diabetes, due to an ageing population, decreased physical activity, and rapidly rising numbers of overweight and obese people (Diabetes UK 2012). Increased longevity in people with diabetes is due to better cardiovascular risk protection after diagnosis (NICE 2008).

Definition

Diabetes mellitus occurs due to either hypo-secretion of insulin or hypoactivity of insulin, causing blood glucose levels to remain elevated. As a result, the cells are unable to utilise glucose for energy purposes (Marieb & Hoehn 2010).

Main types of diabetes

There are two major types of diabetes: type 1 and type 2. In type 1 diabetes, the pancreas makes little or no insulin because the beta cells in the Islets of Langerhans, which produce insulin, have been destroyed through an autoimmune reaction. Thus, people with type 1 diabetes depend on insulin injections to survive. Type 1 diabetes usually appears before the age of 40 and is the less common of the two main types. It accounts for 10% of all people with diabetes (Diabetes UK 2012).

Type 2 diabetes results from reduced insulin production and reduced tissue sensitivity to insulin. It is a progressive disease in which insulin production declines as the disease progresses (Diabetes UK 2012). The treatment of type 2 diabetes involves controlling the condition through diet and drugs, but may now also be controlled by insulin injections. Other newer treatments, such as the long-acting glucagon-like peptide-1 (GLP-1) analogues (such as liraglutide) are also licensed for use (Whitmore 2010). This type of diabetes usually appears in people over the age of 40, though in South Asian people it often appears after the age of 25.

Type 2 is the more common of the two main types and accounts for 90% of people with diabetes (Diabetes UK 2012).

Risk factors

The risk of developing diabetes depends on a combination of genetic, lifestyle, and environmental factors.

Genetic

- *Type I diabetes:* Although more than 85% of type I diabetes occurs in individuals with no previous first-degree family history, the risk among first-degree relatives is about 15 times higher than in the general population. On average, if both parents have the condition, the risk of developing it is up to 30%.

- *Types 2 diabetes:* There is a complex interplay of genetic and environmental factors in type 2 diabetes. It tends to cluster in families. Where there is diabetes in the family, relatives are between two and six times more likely to develop diabetes than those without diabetes in the family (Diabetes UK 2012).

Ethnicity

Type 2 diabetes is up to six times more common in people of South Asian descent and up to three times more common among people of African-Caribbean origin (Diabetes UK 2012).

Obesity

Obesity is the most potent risk factor for type 2 diabetes. It accounts for 80–85% of the overall risk of developing type 2 diabetes and underlies the current global spread of the condition. Almost two in every three people in the UK are overweight or obese; this accounts for 62% of women and 66% of men (Diabetes UK 2012).

Deprivation

Deprivation is strongly associated with higher levels of obesity, physical inactivity, unhealthy diet, smoking, and poor blood pressure control. All these factors are linked to the risk of diabetes or the risk of complications for those already diagnosed with the condition. The most deprived people in the UK are two-and-a-half times more likely than average to have diabetes at any given age (Diabetes UK 2012).

Gestational

Gestational diabetes is a type of diabetes arising during the second or third trimester and it affects up to 5% of pregnancies in the UK. Women who are overweight or obese are at higher risk of getting gestational diabetes. The lifetime risk of developing type 2 diabetes after having gestational diabetes is 30% (Diabetes UK 2012).

Complications

Prolonged hyperglycaemia can cause macrovascular and microvascular damage and is associated with complications affecting a wide range of body systems. Macrovascular complications relate to vascular disease and include coronary artery disease, increased risks of strokes, and peripheral vascular disease. Diabetes is also associated with dyslipidaemia, in which cholesterol and lipid metabolism is imbalanced.

Microvascular complications affect smaller blood vessels in the body such as the kidneys. Indeed, diabetic nephropathy is a leading cause of end-stage renal failure. Of particular significance, however, is the microvascular damage sustained by the small retinal blood vessels in the eyes, leading to the onset of diabetic retinopathy and consequent sight loss. A more detailed account of the capillary degeneration in diabetic retinopathy is provided in a discussion of its pathogenesis (see below).

Diabetic retinopathy

Diabetic retinopathy is one of the leading causes of blindness in the Western world, particularly in individuals of working age. It is a major cause of blindness in people with diabetes (Riordan-Eva & Whitcher 2008).

Risk factors

Risk factors for the development and progression of retinopathy include chronic hyperglycaemia, hypertension, hypercholesterolaemia and smoking (Riordan-Eva & Whitcher 2008). The incidence of diabetic retinopathy is related primarily to duration and control of diabetes and occurs in individuals with a long history of poorly controlled diabetes (Kanski & Bowling 2011). After 20 years from the onset of this condition, more than 60% of those with type 2 diabetes will have diabetic retinopathy, with the presence of maculopathy being the major cause of central visual loss (NICE 2008).

Classification

Diabetic retinopathy can be classified into non-proliferative retinopathy, maculopathy, and proliferative retinopathy. James & Bron (2011) have usefully classified diabetic retinopathy according to the stage reached and the presenting clinical features (see Table 5.1, page 89).

Pathogenesis

Diabetic retinopathy is a progressive microangiopathy characterised by small vessel damage and occlusion (Riordan-Eva & Whitcher 2008). The earliest pathological changes take place in the structural components of the retinal capillaries, where a thickening of the capillary endothelial basement membrane and a reduction in the number of pericytes become apparent. The walls of the capillaries weaken, resulting in the formation of aneurysms. The aneurysms then rupture, causing haemorrhage and the scattering of lipids. The haemorrhages are flame-shaped because of their location within the horizontally oriented nerve fibre layer (see Figure 5.1, page 90).

With the subsequent closing down of new blood vessels, ischaemia and micro infarction of retinal tissue occur, leading to sight loss. The generalised ischaemia results in neovascularisation with consequent haemorrhaging, scar tissue formation and possible retinal detachment (Riordan-Eva & Whitcher 2008). However, maculopathy is the major cause of visual loss for people with type 2 diabetes.

Table 5.1: Classification of diabetic retinopathy

Stage	Description
No retinopathy	There are no abnormal signs present in the retina. Vision is normal.
Background	Microvascular leakage of haemorrhage and exudate away from the macula. Vision is normal.
Maculopathy	Exudate and haemorrhage within the macular region, and/or evidence of retinal oedema, and/or evidence of retinal ischaemia. Vision may be reduced and this condition is sight-threatening.
Pre-proliferative	Evidence of occlusion ('cotton wool spots'). The veins become irregular and may show loops. Vision is normal.
Proliferative	Growth of new blood vessels either on the optic disc or elsewhere on the retina. Vision is affected and it is sight-threatening.
Advanced	The proliferative changes may result in bleeding into the vitreous or between the vitreous and the retina. The retina may also be pulled away from its underlying pigment epithelium (retinal detachment) by a fibrous proliferation associated with the growth of new vessels. Vision is reduced, often acutely with vitreous haemorrhage, and is sight-threatening.

(Adapted from James & Bron 2011)

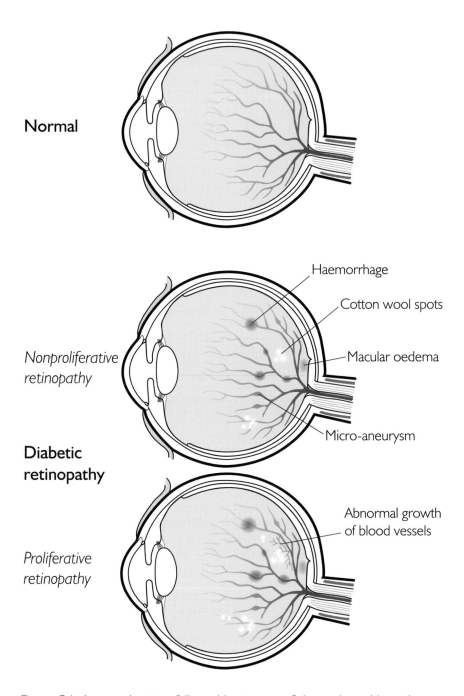

Normal

Haemorrhage

Cotton wool spots

Nonproliferative
retinopathy

Macular oedema

**Diabetic
retinopathy**

Micro-aneurysm

Proliferative
retinopathy

Abnormal growth
of blood vessels

*Figure 5.1: A normal retina, followed by images of the early and late changes
that occur in diabetic retinopathy*

Diabetic maculopathy

Diabetic maculopathy shows itself as a focal or diffuse retinal thickening or oedema, caused by a breakdown of the inner blood-retinal barrier at the level of the retinal capillary endothelium. This allows leakage of fluid and plasma constituents into the surrounding retina. It is more common in type 2 diabetes and requires treatment once it becomes significant, which is defined as any retinal thickening within 500 microns of the fovea, hard exudates within 500 microns of the fovea associated with retinal thickening, or retinal thickening greater than one disc diameter in size, of which any part lies within one disc diameter of the fovea (Riordan-Eva & Whitcher 2008).

Investigations

Imaging plays an increasingly important role in the classification of diabetic retinopathy and therefore needs to reflect the rapid technological advances that are currently taking place.

Digital photography

Digital photography has become the mainstream technology for documenting the presence of diabetic retinopathy and is the method of choice for retinal screening. Colour photography is best used to demonstrate the presence of white lesions such as exudate and cotton wool spots. All other lesions can be most effectively visualised using red-free images. Although most features can be ascertained, intra-retinal microvascular anomalies can only be confidently documented if the nerve fibre layer is also visible (RCO 2012).

Intravenous fluorescein angiography

Fluorescein angiography has had an important role in demonstrating the presence of subtle new-vessel formation and guiding laser, particularly macular laser for oedema and fill-in laser for proliferative retinopathy. Only fluorescein angiography can readily demonstrate the extent and location of capillary dropout. However, the use of fluorescein angiography is waning, with the advent of optical coherence tomography (OCT) and anti-VEGF medications (RCO 2012).

Optical coherence tomography

OCT complements the understanding of maculopathy and highlights the shortcomings of only performing a slit-lamp examination for the purpose of identifying retinal thickening and intra-retinal oedema (RCO 2012).

This technology has also revolutionised the identification of macular oedema, though it is limited by its inability to identify the source of leakage and degree of capillary dropout present. It is particularly suited to determining whether retinal fluid is centre involving or not, which is helpful when selecting patients who are best suited for laser (extrafoveal).

Fluorescein angiography may still be necessary in some cases to guide treatment –

for example, in cases of juxtafoveal leakage and retinal thickening (cyst formation). OCT will also reveal the presence of haemorrhage, exudate and photoreceptor atrophy, which can be enhanced by colour photography. OCT is very useful in assessing vitreo-retinal interface at the macula in differentiating vitreo retinal attachment from vitreo retinal traction, such as vitreo macular traction (RCO 2012).

Retinal screening

The early detection and treatment of diabetic retinopathy is essential because detectable changes occur in the retina before vision is affected. Identifying such changes and providing appropriate treatment will usually prevent permanent visual loss (Riordan-Eva & Whitcher 2008).

Retinal screening is therefore an effective means of detecting diabetic retinopathy as early as possible. Currently, all adults and children aged 12 and over with diabetes (types 1 and 2) are offered annual screening appointments. Screening may be provided in a variety of locations, including primary care surgeries, hospitals and opticians' practices (UK National Screening Committee 2011).

Bentley et al. (2011) suggest that retinal screening offers multiple opportunities for patient education and health promotion to empower patients to take control of their diabetes. It is therefore essential that patients attending retinal screening are educated to understand the importance of attending for annual ophthalmic assessments.

The UK National Screening Committee's classification is aimed at detecting the level of retinopathy to meet standards for referral for ophthalmology specialist opinion and laser treatment option (UK National Screening Committee 2011). This system is used for population screening. The simple classification approach grades the level of retinopathy based on features that retinal screeners (non-ophthalmologists) might be faced with.

This classification identifies four main fundus disease presentations: retinopathy; maculopathy; photocoagulation; and unclassifiable, unobtainable/ungradable.

Current approaches to treatment

Treatment options for diabetic retinopathy include laser photocoagulation for focal and diffuse maculopathy, and proliferative retinopathy. Vitrectomy is performed for persistent vitreous haemorrhage and tractional retinal detachment involving the macula. However, guidelines stress that the risk of visual impairment and blindness can be substantially reduced by a care programme combining methods of early detection with effective treatment of diabetic retinopathy (NICE 2009).

Screening and treatment of diabetic retinopathy will not eliminate all cases of sight loss but can play an important role in substantially reducing the number of patients who will experience sight loss as a result of this condition.

Clinical management and the role of the health and social care professional

Communication and patient-centred care

Management of diabetic retinopathy involves the same approach to self-care as the medical condition to which it is directly attributable. Advice should be given according to the perceived needs and preferences of older people and their families and carers. Older people with type 2 diabetes should have the opportunity to make informed decisions about their care and treatment in partnership with healthcare professionals. Similarly, with the older person's agreement, families and carers should also have the opportunity to be involved in decisions about treatment and care (NICE 2009).

Good communication between the older person and the health and social care professional is essential. This should include the provision of evidence-based information about the condition itself, and its treatment, tailored to meet the older person's needs. Families and carers should also be given the information and support they need (NICE 2009).

Health education

Health education is an important preventative strategy that can be implemented by the health and social care professional when managing older people with diabetic retinopathy. It is important to review the older patient's diabetic control and record their blood pressure. Health education should include the best available research evidence to assist patients in making decisions about lifestyle changes and gain control over the management of their condition. Microvascular complications may be prevented, or their onset delayed, by appropriate medical treatment (Kanski & Bowling 2011).

Making lifestyle changes

When offering advice to older people with type 2 diabetes, healthcare professionals should emphasise the benefits of a healthy balanced diet. Eating high-fibre, low-glycaemic-index sources of carbohydrate (such as fruit, vegetables, wholegrains and pulses) should be encouraged. Low-fat dairy products and oily fish are beneficial. It is important to control the intake of foods containing saturated and trans-fatty acids. Dietary advice can also be integrated with other aspects of lifestyle modification such as guidance on increasing physical activity and losing weight.

Blood glucose control

The health and social care professional should provide older patients and their families with reliable evidence-based information and advice about the importance of maintaining good blood glucose control. Levels of blood glucose should preferably remain below HbAlc 6.5–7.5%, according to the individual's target (NICE 2009). This target is based on the risk of macrovascular and microvascular complications. Older people with type 2 diabetes need to have an ongoing structured evaluation every two to six months to assess their risk factor. A reduction in the prevalence of diabetic retinopathy is associated with tighter blood glucose control (NICE 2009).

Blood pressure management

Effective blood pressure management is as significant as blood glucose control in reducing the risk of progression of diabetic retinopathy in people with type 2 diabetes (UK Prospective Diabetes Study Group 2004). Good blood pressure control is considered to be at or below 140/80mmHg, or in the case of an older person with eye, kidney or cardiovascular damage, at or below 130/80mmHg (NICE 2009). If blood pressure levels consistently exceed these recommended levels, lifestyle advice concerning diet and exercise should be offered as previously outlined (NICE 2009). Older people should be encouraged to adhere to prescribed anti-hypertensive treatment, as diabetic patients with hypertension have a poor visual prognosis (NICE 2009).

Control of lipid levels

Similarly, older people need to comply with drug therapy to reduce serum cholesterol levels, as elevated levels are associated with an increased severity of retinal hard exudate, resulting in decreased visual acuity (NICE 2009).

Value of psychosocial theory

As an effective health educator (Seewoodhary & Watkinson 2011), the health and social care professional needs a good knowledge of psychosocial theory in order to encourage and motivate older people with diabetes to adhere to prescribed treatment, make the necessary lifestyle changes and gain control over their diabetes.

Psychosocial theories attempt to explain the effects of different variables on an individual's health-related behaviour. Such variables include individual health beliefs and attitudes, family attitudes and influence, religious beliefs, social standing, self-esteem, confidence, motivation, depression, and locus of control. Some of the most useful and appropriate psychosocial theories are embodied in the Health Belief Model (Becker 1974), incorporating Bandura's concept of self-efficacy (1977), the Health Action Model (Tones et al. 1990), and Social Learning theory (Rotter 1954). Knowledge and understanding of such models may facilitate more effective promotion of eye health.

Within the domain of public health education, the nurse's role in promoting eye health remains significant, especially with reference to diabetes mellitus. Establishing a therapeutic relationship and providing quality time are essential in building up self-belief and confidence to allow the older person to gain control over the long-term management of diabetes and diabetic retinopathy (Seewoodhary & Watkinson 2011).

Health beliefs and attitudes

Health beliefs and attitudes appear to have a significant influence on whether or not a person will listen to advice and comply with a suggested management strategy. The Health Belief Model (Becker 1974) may be relevant when managing the older person with diabetic retinopathy. This model suggests that a person's decision to modify their beliefs and change their behaviour will be influenced by their evaluation of the feasibility of the suggested treatment or management plan, and the benefits weighed against the costs (a cost-benefit analysis). It is therefore important to explore with the older person their perceptions of diabetes and diabetic retinopathy to determine how much knowledge and understanding they have of these medical conditions.

It is equally important to assess the older person's perception of the likelihood of the diabetic retinopathy becoming more severe, balanced against their perception of the efficacy of making lifestyle changes to gain better control of the diabetes and thus prevent or slow down loss of vision in the longer term. The fear of losing sight is known to promote adherence to treatment in many instances (RNIB 2007). Encouraging self-belief is therefore important, as individuals must believe they are capable of making the required changes in their behaviour (Bandura 1977). If they feel threatened by the prospect of a reduced sighted quality of life, they become incentivised to accept the reality of the threat and make the changes required to manage the situation (Seewoodhary & Watkinson 2011).

Taking individual responsibility

A key objective for the health and social care professional managing older people with diabetic retinopathy is to increase their motivation to take responsibility for maintaining control of the diabetes by making the necessary lifestyle changes and commit to an ongoing retinal screening programme. The Health Action model (Tones et al. 1990) identifies self-esteem as a key component in the motivation system. Self-perception is a major influence on an individual's readiness to take a health decision.

The central concept is perceived control, which is a mediating factor in behaviour developed from social learning theory (Rotter 1954). In exploring the health beliefs and attitudes of the older person with diabetic retinopathy, a knowledge and understanding of social learning theory may help health and social care professionals to appreciate the ways in which individuals explain what has happened to them and the situations they have found themselves in. This will in turn help to determine their locus of control as internal or external, and provide a rationale for the most appropriate approach to take to promote or maintain their motivation. Individuals with an internal locus of control believe they are responsible for their own health. Those individuals with an external locus of control believe that their decisions and actions are limited by external factors, such as powerful others, chance, fate, or luck (Rotter 1954), and consequently abrogate their responsibilities.

Importantly, in trying to increase motivation, older patients with diabetic retinopathy should be encouraged to get involved as much as possible with their own care and management, particularly those who believe they are powerless to take any action. If they are encouraged to participate in making decisions about their own situation, this helps strengthen their adherence to prescribed treatment and suggested management strategies. Clearly, health and social care professionals have a duty of care to contribute to patient education and motivate family members alike. However, it is only through empowerment that older patients can begin to learn about their diabetes and associated ocular problems and thus take responsibility for adherence and self-caring.

The psychological role

The diagnosis of diabetes can be psychologically devastating for an older person and may trigger the onset of depression. Indeed, depression is the most common psychiatric disorder in the diabetes community (Diabetes UK 2012) and is associated with worse diabetes outcomes (Raval et al. 2010). Depression can have a serious impact on a person's well-being and their ability and motivation to self-manage their condition (Diabetes UK 2012). Raval et al. (2010) showed that patients with depression and diabetes had poorer self-management and poor adherence to anti-diabetic, lipid-lowering and anti-hypertensive treatment. They were also more likely to have higher cardiovascular risk factors such as smoking, obesity, sedentary lifestyle, and uncontrolled hyperglycaemia (Raval et al. 2010). Patients with depression and diabetes are more likely to have higher macrovascular and microvascular complications and higher mortality rates (Raval et al. 2010).

More significantly, depression is also associated with a higher incidence of diabetic retinopathy among adults with type 2 diabetes. Thus, improving the treatment of depression in patients with diabetes could contribute to the prevention of diabetic retinopathy (Sieu et al. 2011). Clearly, by addressing depression, glycaemic control is enhanced, and mood and quality of life are significantly improved (Diabetes UK 2012). It is therefore important to provide ongoing psychological support to older patients and their families in order to address the depression, maintain self-esteem and improve self-management of the diabetes (Watkinson & Seewoodhary 2008).

Inevitably, any visual impairment arising from the diabetic retinopathy may compound the older person's inability to manage both the diabetes and depression, due to loss of motivation and self-management skills. This in turn has psychosocial and economic implications.

Future perspectives

The discussion so far has shown that diabetes mellitus and its complications, especially diabetic retinopathy, will be an economic health burden for the UK in the future. Unfortunately, there will be limited resources available to deal with these issues in the coming years, due to predicted financial restraints. Sadly, older people with diabetic retinopathy will also experience the economic and psychological burdens of visual impairment or sight loss due to diabetic retinopathy. Reducing or averting such burdens involves individuals taking responsibility for making decisive changes in favour of healthier lifestyles. Thus, effective delivery of public health information about diabetes to all age groups remains crucially important in trying to maintain quality of life in older age.

At present, laser treatment is the only proven treatment for the changes caused by diabetic retinopathy. Laser treatment for macular changes is not as successful as that for proliferative retinopathy but does prevent serious sight loss in 60% to 70% of cases. Recently, there have been some significant advances in the treatment of diabetic macular oedema. As this remains an area of active research, it is likely that other new therapeutic options will become available over the next few years (RCO 2012). Clearly, there is evidence to support the benefits of photocoagulation using the modified Early Treatment Diabetic Retinopathy Study (ETDRS) protocol versus no treatment, or compared to mild modified grid laser. There is also emerging evidence to suggest that similar outcomes can be achieved with sub-threshold micro-pulse diode laser therapy (RCO 2012).

Overall, photocoagulation treatment reduces the risk of visual loss and works over a long timescale, but it is clear that recovery of vision is much harder to achieve using laser treatment alone, particularly in patients with more severe macular oedema (RCO 2012).

Current treatments using intra-vitreal anti-VEGF agents such as Lucentis (ranibizumab) and Avastin, with prompt or delayed focal laser photocoagulation, are most effective in preserving and restoring vision when centre-involved macular oedema is present and acuity is reduced to 20/32 or less (RCO 2012). Several other clinical trials are currently assessing the use of ranibizumab in the treatment of diabetic macular oedema, and we are awaiting the results of these studies. Work is also underway to develop methods of slowly releasing anti-VEGF treatment from within the eye (RCO 2012).

Such new treatments represent a positive approach to treating diabetic macular oedema for the future. At the same time, they must be supported by good control of diabetes, including monitoring blood glucose, blood pressure and lipid levels, weight, exercise and providing help with smoking cessation (Diabetes UK 2012).

Conclusion

In summary, this chapter has focused on managing older people with diabetic retinopathy. As diabetic retinopathy is one of the significant complications of diabetes mellitus, an overview of this metabolic disease was initially provided, covering its epidemiology, main types, risk factors, blood glucose regulation and main complications.

This was followed by an overview of diabetic retinopathy, including its risk factors, classification, pathogenesis and investigations. Retinal screening was presented as one of the key ways of detecting the early changes caused by diabetic retinopathy, in order to provide appropriate treatment to arrest further development of the condition. Current approaches to treatment were then explored, before a detailed discussion of the role of the health and social care professional in managing the care of older people with diabetic retinopathy. Future perspectives were subsequently covered, with specific reference to the future use of anti-VEGF agents in the treatment of macular oedema, before drawing some overall conclusions.

Having addressed the four major age-related ocular diseases, the next chapter presents some of the external ocular conditions commonly experienced by older people.

References

Bandura, A. (1977). *Social Learning Theory.* Englewood Cliff, NJ, USA: Prentice Hall.

Becker, M.H. (ed) (1974). *The Health Belief Model and Personal Health Behaviour.* New Jersey, USA: Slack Inc, Thorofare.

Bentley, P., Gibbons, H. & Mapani, A. (2011). Diabetes and diabetic retinopathy. *International Journal of Ophthalmic Practice.* **2** (4), 181–86.

Diabetes UK (2014). What is diabetes? www.diabetes.org.uk/Guide-to-diabetes/What-is-diabetes (Last accessed: 22 April 2014).

James, B. & Bron, A. (2011). *Lecture Notes on Ophthalmology.* 11th edn. Oxford: Wiley-Blackwell.

Kanski, J. & Bowling, B. (2011). *Clinical Ophthalmology: A Systematic Approach.* 7th edn. London: Elsevier.

Marieb, E. & Hoehn, K. (2010). *Human Anatomy and Physiology.* 8th edn. London: Pearson.

UK National Screening Committee (2011). www.diabeticeye.screening.nhs.uk/ (Last accessed: 24 April 2014).

National Institute for Health and Clinical Excellence (2008). *Type 2 diabetes. The management of type 2 diabetes. Clinical Guideline 66.* London: NICE. http:/www.nice.org.uk/nicemedia/pdf/cg66niceguideline.pdf (Last accessed: 1 August 2013).

National Institute for Health and Clinical Excellence (2009). *Type 2 diabetes. The management of type 2 diabetes. Clinical Guideline 87.* London: NICE. http://www.nice.org.uk/nicemedia/live/12165/44320/44320.pdf (Last accessed: 1 August 2013).

Raval, A., Dhanaraj, E., Bhansali, A., Grover, S. & Tiwari, P. (2010). Prevalence and determinants of depression in type 2 diabetes patients in a tertiary care centre. *Indian Journal of Medical Research.* **132**, 195–200.

Riordan-Eva, P. & Whitcher, J. (2008). *Vaughan and Asbury's General Ophthalmology.* 17th edn. New York, USA: Lange Medical Books/McGraw-Hill.

Rotter, J.B. (1954). *Social Learning and Clinical Psychology.* Englewood Cliff, NJ, USA: Prentice Hall.

Royal College of Ophthalmologists (2012). *Diabetic Retinopathy Guidelines 2012 (Minor update July 2013).* London: RCO. www.rcophth.ac.uk/page.asp?section=451&sectiontitle=Clinical (Last accessed: 30 July 2013).

Royal National Institute of Blind People (2007). *Older People and Eye Tests: Don't Let Age Rob You of Your Sight.* www.optical.org/goc/download.cfm?docid=13D79738-B2EC-4C44. (Last accessed: 24 April 2014).

Seewoodhary, R. & Watkinson, S. (2011). Public health knowledge of glaucoma: implications for the ophthalmic nurse. *International Journal of Ophthalmic Practice.* **2** (4), 170–77.

Sieu, N., Katon, W., Lin, E.H., Russo, J., Ludman, E. & Ciechanowski, P. (Sept–Oct 2011). Depression and incident diabetic retinopathy: a prospective cohort study. *General Hospital Psychiatry.* **33** (5), 429–35.

Tones, B.K., Tilford, S. & Keeley Robinson, Y. (1990). *Health Education: Effectiveness and Efficiency.* London: Chapman and Hall.

UK Prospective Diabetes Study Group (2004). Risk of progression of retinopathy and vision loss related to tight blood pressure control in type 2 diabetes mellitus. *Archives of Ophthalmology.* **122** (11), 1631–40.

Watkinson, S. & Seewoodhary, R. (2008). Ocular complications associated with diabetes mellitus. *Nursing Standard.* **22** (27), 51–57.

Whitmore, C. (2010). Type 2 diabetes and obesity in adults. *British Journal of Nursing.* **19** (14), 880–86.

Chapter 6

Common external eye disorders in older people

Mahesh Seewoodhary and Cecilia Awelewa

This chapter covers

- Introduction
- Dry eyes
- Lid mal-positioning disorders
- Blepharitis
- Conclusion

Introduction

This chapter discusses three common extra-ocular disorders in older people, which pose a potential threat to sight: dry eyes, lid mal-positioning (ectropion and entropion), and blepharitis. For each type of disorder, the pathophysiology, management and nursing care will be discussed. In older people, the immune system becomes less active, and this can lead to eye infection or inflammation.

Vision is the most important sense we have. Loss of vision can isolate a person, and fear of blindness is more common in older people presenting in ophthalmic units (Vafidis 2007). Around 1 in 5 people aged 75 and above have experienced sight loss (RNIB 2012); and eye problems account for more than 6% of all accident and emergency attendances (Marsden 2002). It is essential that healthcare practitioners recognise these problems in older people and take appropriate action to prevent sight loss (Watkinson & Seewoodhary 2007).

Older people are also more likely to suffer ill-health (NMC 2009b), and may present with challenges such as poor dexterity, mobility, memory loss, anxieties, fears and depression. These challenges need to be addressed to ensure that older people are empowered when they attend eye units. Ophthalmic healthcare practitioners must follow the principles laid out in the NMC guidance for care of older people (2009). These principles will ensure that older people are cared for in a dignified and compassionate manner.

Dry eyes

Dry eye is a common problem. It ranges in severity from mildly irritating to severely disabling (Tornquist 2012). It is associated with a rise in osmolality of the tear film and inflammation of the ocular surface. In the past, dry eye disease was considered an irreversible, inevitable change due to age (Henderson 2013). Inflammation plays a key role in dry eye, and anti-inflammatory treatment can both improve the ocular surface and prevent disease progression. The incidence of dry eye ranges from 3% to 15% in patients aged 50 years and older (Schaumberg et al. 2009). The rate increases with age, from 10.7% in subjects aged 48 to 59 years, to 17.9% in those older than 80 (Tornquist 2012). Although dry eye is common worldwide it remains an under-recognised problem; and it does affect the older person's quality of life (Smith 2007).

Pathophysiology of dry eye syndrome

Dry eye syndrome is defined as a multifactorial disease of the tears and ocular surface that results in symptoms of discomfort, visual disturbance, tear film instability and potential damage to the ocular surface (Dry Eye Workshop Report 2007, Henderson 2013). Tears are a complex secretion derived from the lacrimal gland, the tarsal glands and the conjunctival goblet cells (Seewoodhary & Watkinson 2009). They play a key role in lubricating the conjunctival and corneal epithelial cells as well as preventing infections. This is because tears carry protective antibodies and antibacterial agents such as lysozyme, lactoferrin and immunoglobulin. A healthy tear film provides a smooth optical refracting surface for the eye and prevents corneal dryness (Riordan-Eva & Whitcher 2008).

The tear film consists of three distinct layers (see Figure 6.1, page 103):

1. Outer lipid layer
2. Middle watery layer
3. Innermost mucin layer

Two major mechanisms have been implicated in the pathophysiology of dry eye disease: inflammation and hyperosmolarity (Henderson 2013).

According to Henderson (2013), measuring inflammation has remained a difficult task in ophthalmic practice. Tears hyperosmolarity is easily measured in the laboratory and is a better indicator of dry eye tests when compared with Schirmers test tear breakup time of staining with dyes (Henderson 2013). Hyperosmolarity is associated with increased saltiness of the tears, which is linked with water deficiency and increased evaporation (Dry Eye Workshop

2007). Tear hyperosmolarity increases cell death in both the cornea and conjunctiva. The destruction of goblet cells is a hallmark of dry eye disease and is also a major contributor to the disease (Henderson 2013). The reflex tearing increases the inflammatory response by releasing inflammatory cytokines. These subsequently stimulate the inflammatory cells and lymphocytes. All these inflammatory responses increase the degeneration and destruction of the goblet cells, and tear film instability, resulting in a vicious circle, as seen in Figures 6.2 and 6.3 (Page 104).

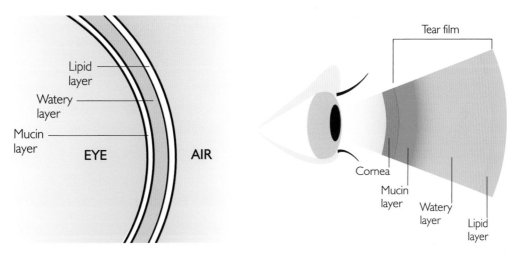

Figure 6.1: The tear film and its relationship to the corneal surface

Two major mechanisms have been implicated in the pathophysiology of dry eye disease: inflammation and hyperosmolarity (Henderson 2013).

According to Henderson (2013), measuring inflammation has remained a difficult task in ophthalmic practice. Tears hyperosmolarity is easily measured in the laboratory and is a better indicator of dry eye tests when compared with Schirmers test tear breakup time of staining with dyes (Henderson 2013). Hyperosmolarity is associated with increased saltiness of the tears, which is linked with water deficiency and increased evaporation (Dry Eye Workshop 2007). Tear hyperosmolarity increases cell death in both the cornea and conjunctiva. The destruction of goblet cells is a hallmark of dry eye disease and is also a major contributor to the disease (Henderson 2013). The reflex tearing increases the inflammatory response by releasing inflammatory cytokines. These subsequently stimulate the inflammatory cells and lymphocytes. All these inflammatory responses increase the degeneration and destruction of the goblet cells, and tear film instability, resulting in a vicious circle, as seen in Figures 6.2 and 6.3 (page 104).

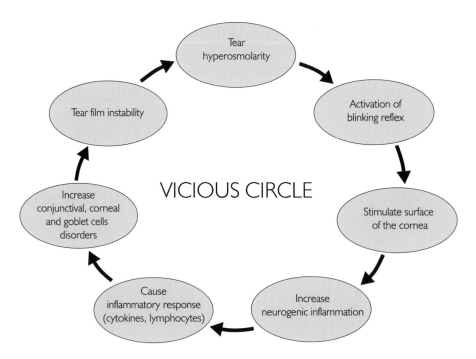

Figure 6.2: The mechanism of the pathophysiology of dry eye disease
(Based on Christophe Baudouin. July 2011)

Inflammation disrupts normal neuronal control of tearing

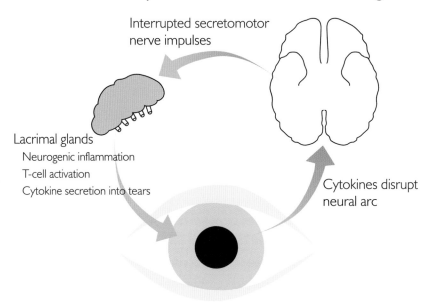

Figure 6.3: The effects of inflammation and its harmful effects on tears

Lam *et al.* (2009) discovered that conjunctival and corneal epithelial cells can be stimulated by abnormalities in the tear film, making them active participants in the inflammatory process, and not just bystander tissues that are injured during the course of the disease. The corneal and conjunctival cells actually produce cytokines and inflammatory mediators that amplify the disease process.

Dry eye disease can take one of two forms (Dry Eye Workshop 2007):

Group 1: Aqueous deficient
Causes include Sjogren's syndrome, systemic drugs, dehydration

Group 2: Evaporative
Causes include low blinking rate, disorders of the eyelids, vitamin A deficiency.

Both types of dry eye disease can also occur in combination and the symptoms can be much worse (Dry Eye Workshop 2007). Another mechanism that may trigger dry eye disease is corneal sensation impairment. A loss of sensory drive to the lacrimal gland may diminish tear secretion, as occurs in Herpes Zoster Ophthalmicus and with overuse of anaesthetic eye drops. Environmental factors may also be responsible for dry eye symptoms. Patients often complain that reading and computer use exacerbate their dry eye symptoms (Schaumberg 2011). Decreased blink rates and rapid tear breakup of the tear film occur during computer use in people with dry eye disease when compared with normal subjects. Bron (2011) presents a triple causal classification of dry eye disease (see Figure 6.4).

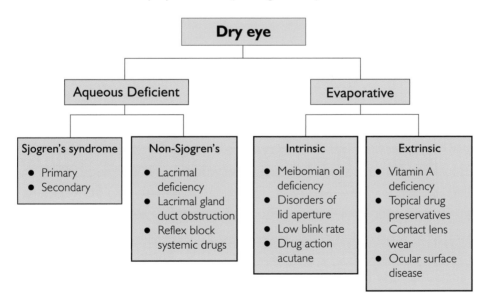

Figure 6.4: Causal classification of dry eye disease
(Adapted from Bron 2011a)

Risk factors for dry eye syndrome include:

- Thyrotoxicosis,
- Sjogren's syndrome
- Blepharitis
- Meibomian gland dysfunction.

Meibomian gland dysfunction appears to to have a higher incidence in the Asian population than in the Caucasian population (Schaumberg 2011).

To guard against a recurrence of dry eye syndrome, lid hygiene is essential and the regime should be continued even after the condition has apparently cleared (Din & Patel 2012). Bacterial lipases will affect the quality of tears and may cause dry eyes secondary to increased ocular surface water evaporation (Sawant & Manoj 2006). Any one of the layers of the tear film can become deficient (Seewoodhary & Watkinson 2009). A lack of mucin leads to poor lubrication of the corneal epithelium and subsequent irritation.

Mucin deficiency is found in trachoma, ocular pemphigoid and avitaminosis A. Lipid deficiencies occur in chronic blepharitis, where secreting cells are scarred. Insufficient lipid formation causes rapid evaporation of the aqueous layer.

Deficiency of the aqueous layer occurs in lacrimal gland excision or in kerato-conjunctivitis Sicca. Symptoms include:

- Burning
- Itching
- Gritty eyes
- Blurred vision.

The older patient will experience these symptoms more frequently in warmer environments, where tear evaporation is highest. Irritants in the atmosphere, such as tobacco smoke, and prolonged reading will worsen the symptoms (Seewoodhary & Watkinson 2009).

Older people with dry eye are at higher risk of eye infection from bacteria, viruses and fungi. Patients presenting with a history of recurrent eye infection should therefore be considered as a suspect dry eye (Seewoodhary & Watkinson 2009). The patient may complain of mucous strands lying in the conjunctival sac. These strands are attached to the corneal epithelium and may cause a recurrent corneal abrasion. The symptoms of pain, redness, blurring of vision and reflex tearing then become acute, prompting the patient to seek emergency treatment.

Diagnosing dry eye

There are four main ways of diagnosing dry eye:

1. The condition is indicated by a tear breakup time of less than 10 seconds. This is assessed using a slit lamp bio-microscope. Rapid tear breakup time leads to more frequent blinking.

2. Schirmer's tear test measurement of less than 10mm in 5 minutes is considered positive.

3. Rose Bengal dye staining of the dead cells of the conjunctiva and cornea is a reliable indication.

4. Slit lamp examination of the anterior segment will reveal lack of tear meniscus on the lid margin, as well as the state of the tear film when stained with fluorescein or when dry cells are stained with Rose Bengal. A close view of the lid margins will help to evaluate meibomian gland dysfunction.

It is recognised that lid disease and meibum alterations contribute to changes in the tear film and the ocular surface (Henderson 2013). Both Figure 6.5 and Figure 6.6 show corneal complications in an older person with dry eye. The fluorescein dye test in Figure 6.6 shows early corneal changes, whereas Figure 6.5 shows a more extensive corneal involvement.

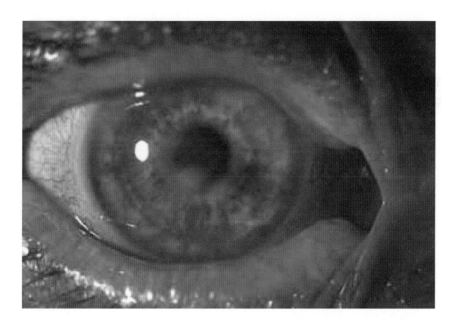

Figure 6.5: Extensive corneal complication
Printed with permission from the Prince Charles Eye Unit, Windsor (2012)

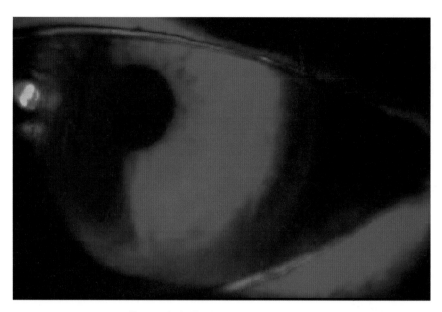

Figure 6.6: Early corneal changes
Printed with permission from the Prince Charles Eye Unit, Windsor (2012)

The patient history often provides useful clues to the causes of dry eye syndrome. For example, the medication history may reveal that the patient is on antidepressants, diuretics, antihistamine, beta blockers or nasal decongestants.

Asbell (2011) stresses that, when examining the eye, ophthalmic practitioners often ignore the lid, the meibomian gland orifices, and the quantity of the expressed meibum, thereby missing an essential aspect of the assessment in patients with ocular surface disease.

Managing patients with dry eyes

There is no cure for the condition so the aim of the treatment is to relieve the patient's discomfort by providing a smooth optical surface and to reduce the risk of serious complications such as infections (Tornquist 2012). Treatment consists of either conserving the tears that are being formed, or adding to them by means of artificial tears. Geerling (2011) says that the majority of patients, regardless of the disease subtype, are initially treated with lubricants because they are widely available. Risk factors must be dealt with to promote comfort and prevent ocular complication (Riordan-Eva & Whitcher 2008). Patients with blepharitis will be instructed by nurses on how to apply warm compresses and maintain lid hygiene (Din & Patel 2012).

The importance of avoiding risk factors or exacerbating conditions, such as certain medications, low-humidity environments and specific head positions during computer use, is explained (Watkinson & Seewoodhary 2007). However, these non-pharmacologic interventions have poor compliance among many patients.

Tears can be conserved temporarily by means of punctal occlusion using gelatine or silicon plugs, or permanently by means of punctal cauterisation. Bron (2011) suggests that a short course of topical steroids is advisable prior to punctal plugs in patients with moderate or severe aqueous-deficient dry eye disease. The rationale is that punctal plugs may not only conserve the tears, but may also conserve inflammatory mediators. Steroids can be helpful initially to damp down the inflammation, and possibly to increase the effectiveness of the plugs. In Figure 6.7, the red arrow shows a silicon plug in puncta.

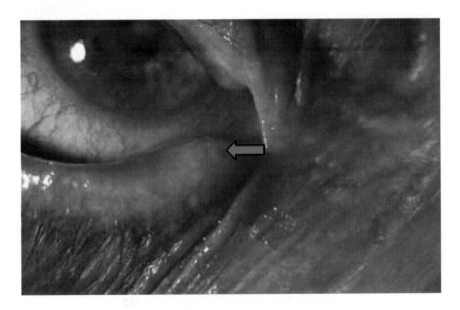

Figure 6.7: Punctal occlusion by silicon plug
Photo printed by permission of the Prince Charles Eye Unit, Windsor (2012)

Tear replacement therapy involves using artificial tears such as Lacri-Lube and hypromellose. Mucolytic agents may also be of value in breaking up the tenacious mucous filaments.

Patients must be encouraged to eat a healthy diet (Sawant & Manoj 2006). Green leafy vegetables, carrots and fruit are good sources of vitamins A, C and E. Vitamins A, C and E are known antioxidants and can protect against dry eyes. Recent studies have shown that essential fatty acids can play a major role in the treatment of dry eyes as well as blepharitis.

An increase in dietary intake of omega-3 fatty acids helps to reduce the inflammation associated with dry eye disease. It also decreases cell apoptosis (Sawant & Manoj 2006). Systemic use of tetracycline derivatives is often prescribed for patients who have developed severe dry eyes due to meibomian gland dysfunction (Geerling 2011). These reduce the proteolytic enzymes in the tears, thus helping to alleviate the symptoms.

Contact lens wear is usually contraindicated in severe dry eyes, as the cornea may become prone to ulceration and scarring. However, the use of bandage contact lenses is beneficial in severe dry eye when other therapy has failed (Tornquist 2012), as this facilitates ocular surface healing. Any allergic reaction to preservatives must be noted and should be avoided.

Artificial tears therapy mainly consists of non-medicated viscous solutions (Moorfields Eye Hospital 2006). When deciding which type of artificial tears to use, there are some important differences between the various products. Carbomer 0.2% eye drops (Liquivisc) and carmellose 1% (Celluvisc) provide ocular lubrication for the relief of dry eyes syndromes associated with tear deficiency (Moorfields Eye Hospital 2006). The following artificial tears are also often prescribed for the relief of dry eyes associated with deficient tear secretions or lubrication of hard or gas-permeable contact lenses. These include hypromellose 0.3%, polyvinyl alcohol 1.4% and sodium hyaluronate 0.1%.

Artificial tears such as polyvinyl alcohol 1.4% (SNO tears) have a long track record and are not likely to cause hypersensitivity. They increase the tear breakup time (Watkinson & Seewoodhary 2008b). Patients who develop hypersensitivity may be prescribed Liquifilm tears, as these are available as preservative-free drops (Moorfields Eye Hospital 2006).

Healthcare professionals must still enquire whether the preservative-free eye drops are causing ocular irritation, as Liquifilm Tears (preservative-free) contain povidone, sodium chloride, sodium hydroxide or hydrochloric acid (Moorfields Eye Hospital 2006).

Any underlying causes must be attended to, such as vitamin A supplements or treatment of thyroid eye disease. The wearing of goggles can provide a local high-humidity environment, thus reducing the loss of fluid through evaporation.

The patient's tears can be measured in the outpatient department using SNO strips. A reading below 5mm in less than 5 minutes would confirm dry eye. If the patient's symptoms are relieved by the appropriate treatment, this must be continued. However, if the patient is not satisfied with the treatment, then the ophthalmologist must explore other treatments (Asbell 2011). Drops that contain preservatives are particularly toxic to the ocular surface. Asbell (2011) suggests that topical cyclosporine is reserved for patients with severe findings. Low-dose steroid medication can also be very effective for many patients with inflammatory ocular surface disease.

Another treatment option approved by the US Food and Drug Administration is hydroxypropyl cellulose insert, which is a tear pellet that is placed in the lower cul-de-sac. The pellet melts with the patient's own tears, providing lubrication over a period of time. This is applied at night, as the lubricant is rather thick and can blur vision during the day.

The overall aims include:

- Lessening of the patient's symptoms
- Lengthening of tear breakup time
- Reduction in the areas of Rose Bengal staining (the dry spots)
- Avoidance of serious complications such as permanently damaged cornea and loss of visual acuity resulting from infections
- Improving the patient's quality of life.

Should infection occur, it should be treated with topical antibiotic. Dry eyes are troublesome eyes with potential to blindness. The international Dry Eye Workshop (DEW), held in 2007, has successfully achieved its aims of giving health practitioners a better understanding of the complexities of dry eye disease.

Following the DEW Report, it is recommended that healthcare practitioners educate patients about care management of dry eyes. Nevertheless, Asbell (2011) says that there remains an under-appreciation of dry eye disease by both European and US health professionals. Dry eye disease can negatively affect patient quality of vision as well as comfort (Smith 2007). The earlier dry eye disease is diagnosed and managed, the lower the chance of serious problems developing (Seewoodhary & Watkinson 2009).

Practical nursing considerations

When managing the care of older patients with dry eye disease, the following principles should be considered (Watkinson & Seewoodhary 2007):

- The older patient must be thoroughly assessed, and the findings documented. For example, history taking, visual acuity recording and an eye examination under slit lamp must be carried out.
- The nurse must check if older people are able to instil their drops by assessing their dexterity. Drop aid may be advised if necessary. A plan of care must be formulated to evaluate progress.
- If the older patient is from a minority ethnic group, the nurse will provide individualised care, which may involve family members to promote understanding of the needs of this age group.

- Relevant health information is given, such as use of artificial tears to promote ocular comfort, healthy eating, and regular attendance at an eye clinic. Improving the home environment, avoiding smoky and polluted atmospheres are very important . Information leaflets on dry eyes and related eye disorders (such as blepharitis) must be provided and discussed with the patient.

- Documentation of nursing interventions must be evident in the patient notes.

- In the interest of hygiene and safety, the older person should follow correct hand-washing guidelines before instilling eye medications.

- Advice should be given about driving hazards if vision is not clear due to tear deficiency or use of ointment.

- The nurse is professionally responsible for providing a high standard of patient care. The patient's dignity and confidentiality must be maintained at all times. The Nursing and Midwifery Council code plays a vital role in guiding best practice and patient-centred care (NMC 2008).

- The importance of healthy eating, as part of care management of dry eye, should be reinforced at each visit.

The philosophy of care for older people with dry eye is to encourage self-caring and concordance with treatment and long-term management. The psychosocial care of the patient must also be addressed, as depression is often linked with dry eye diseases in older people. Appropriate referral must be made to relevant agencies for collaborative care such as counsellors and pharmacists (Standing 2011).

Dry eye management is rewarding in older people. The ophthalmic nurse's role is vital in patient assessment and education. Dry eye remains a threat to vision but it can be prevented. In this age group, dry eye syndrome must be managed effectively by all relevant team members. Improving staff knowledge will make a difference to the quality of patient care and prevention of sight loss.

Lid mal-positioning disorders

Ageing is known to affect the structure and function of the eyelid (Riordan-Eva & Whitcher 2008). This can be a threat to vision if not managed at an early stage. The eyelid protects the eye by preventing contact with foreign materials and preventing excessive dryness of the cornea and conjunctiva (Pavan-Langston 2007). Figure 6.8 (page 113) shows the lid position against the globe and its various anatomical landmarks.

The palpebral fissure must be wide enough to allow light to enter the pupil, and should close sufficiently to provide protection and moisture to the globe. The lid contours and palpebral fissures should be symmetrical in order to avoid cosmetic deformity (Pavan-Langston 2007).

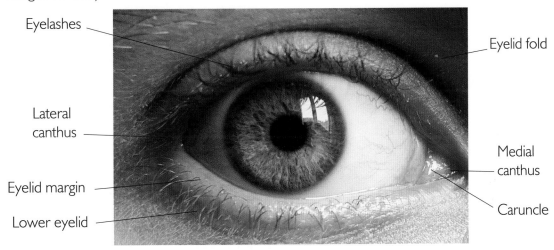

Figure 6.8: The lid position against the globe
(Photo printed with permission from the Prince Charles Eye Unit, Windsor 2012)

A cross-sectional view can be seen in Figure 6.9. This shows that the eyelids are lamellar structures covered on their outer surfaces by skin and on their inner surfaces by conjunctiva. In between are the fibrous tarsal plates, the orbital septum, the levator muscle, the Muller's muscle, the lower lid retractors and the orbicularis muscle. The lids and the palpebral fissures are maintained in a stable position by periosteal attachments provided by the medial and lateral canthal tendons. The closure of the eye is by the orbicularis muscle, which is supplied by the seventh cranial nerve (Riordan-Eva & Whitcher 2008).

Pathophysiology of ectropion

An ectropion (see Figure 6.10, page 115) is defined as a mal-position of the eyelid in which the lid margin is turned away from the globe (Kanski & Bowling 2011). The lower lid is involved much more commonly than the upper one. This is caused by laxity and degenerative changes in the orbicularis muscle. In health, this muscle is circular and has various attachments with the lid margin to ensure close apposition with the globe (Pavan-Langston 2008).

There are two types of ectropion, as seen in Table 6.1 (page 115).

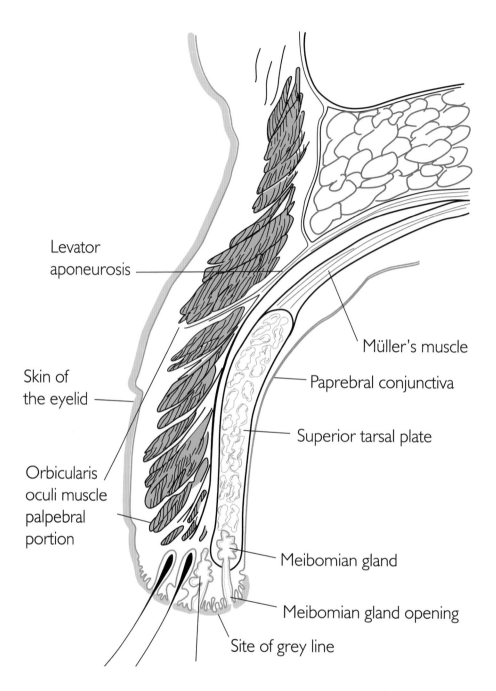

Levator
aponeurosis

Skin of
the eyelid

Orbicularis
oculi muscle
palpebral
portion

Müller's muscle

Paprebral conjunctiva

Superior tarsal plate

Meibomian gland

Meibomian gland opening

Site of grey line

Figure 6.9: A cross-section of the eyelid

Table 6.1: Congenital and acquired ectropion

Congenital	Very uncommon and is found with blepharophimosis. Lid eversion is minimal, so treatment is rarely required.
Acquired: Involutional	Age-related due to laxity of the orbicularis muscle, and attenuation of lower lid retractors and canthal tendon. Treatment is surgical by surgical correction.
Paralytic	This occurs due to facial palsy or trauma to the nerve and muscle.
Mechanical	Caused by large lesions that push or pull the lid away from the eye. Treatment is surgical and is aimed towards removing the lesion.
Cicatricial	This is caused by scarring associated with skin traction and tissue loss. Treatment is surgical correction and skin graft.

(Adapted from Pavan-Langston 2008)

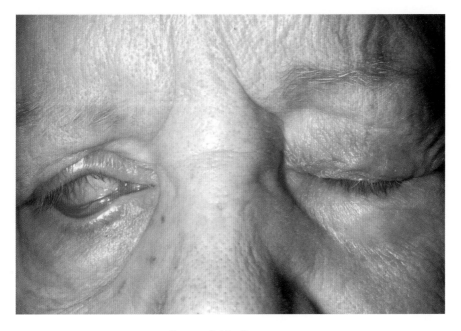

Figure 6.10: Ectropion

The symptoms of ectropion include:

● Constant watery eye

● Irritation

● Redness

● Discomfort.

The cornea is at risk of ulceration. If left untreated, sight can be threatened by corneal damage (Kanski 2007).

Pathophysiology of entropion

An entropion is a mal-position of the eyelid in which the lid margin is turned inwards towards the eye (Riordan-Eva & Whitcher 2008). The condition is illustrated in Figure 6.11. Entropion can damage the cornea because the eyelashes turn in, resulting in keratitis and ulceration.

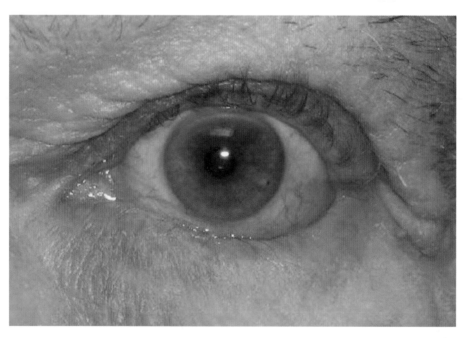

Figure 6.11: A patient with entropion
(Photo printed with permission from the Prince Charles Eye Unit, Windsor, 2012)

The pathology is caused by involutional changes of the eyelid structure, causing the tarsal plate to become soft and the orbicularis muscle to go into spasms (Pavan-Langston 2008).

There are two types of entropion, as shown in Table 6.2 (opposite).

Table 6.2: Congenital and acquired entropion

Congenital	Usually associated with other ocular abnormalities such as tarsal hypoplasia or microphthalmia. Mild cases resolve spontaneously. Surgery is reserved if this is severe.
Acquired: Involutional	This is age-related, involving the lower lid in which the orbicularis muscle goes into spasms. Treated with surgical correction.
Spastic	This is temporary or intermittent accentuation of the involutional changes caused by irritation and vigorous lid closure. Treatment is aimed at removing the cause of irritation or surgically correcting the lower eyelid.
Cicatricial	This is due to tarsoconjunctival shrinkage. Common causes include trachoma, Steven-Johnson syndrome, and pemphigus, mechanical, thermal or chemical injury.
	Treatment may consist of marginal rotation of the lid margin and grafts of mucosa to replace contracted tarsus and conjunctiva.

(Adapted from Pavan-Langston 2008)

The symptoms of entropion include:

● Pain

● Foreign body feelings

● Watery eyes

● Ocular discomfort.

Managing older patients with ectropion and entropion

Both entropion and ectropion are a severe threat to sight and must be managed in a dedicated eye unit by an ophthalmologist and nurses with specialist knowledge and qualifications (Marsden 2007). The patient will be assessed holistically and their visual acuity recorded. A thorough slit lamp eye examination will be carried out to assess the anterior segment. Fluorescein dye will be used to stain the outer segment. The extent of corneal damage will then be assessed and documented. Keeping accurate documentation of the eye is important for medico-legal reasons (NMC 2008). The patient will be instructed to keep the eyelid clean. In the case of patients with entropion, the lower eyelid will be taped down on the cheek to prevent the lashes from scratching the cornea. An appointment will be given to attend the eye clinic or surgery. Antibiotic eye drops or ointment will be prescribed by the ophthalmologist if the cornea has become compromised, or if an infection is present. Artificial tear drops will also be prescribed to promote ocular comfort.

Practical nursing considerations

When managing the care of older people with ectropion and entropion, it is important to assess each patient holistically and plan their care accordingly (Smith & Field 2011), bearing the following points in mind:

- The care must be always be patient-centred (Standing 2011).

- The ophthalmic nurse must be able to make clinical judgements and take appropriate action for the older patient, ensuring that they work to a high standard and within the remit of the NMC code of practice (NMC 2008).

- A holistic approach is essential with older people, as many of them have difficulty hearing clearly, and many are anxious and worried about their sight.

- The medication history must be clearly documented, especially if the older patient is on aspirin or warfarin.

- Hospital policies and clinical governance guidelines to ensure patient safety and well-being must be followed.

- Relevant information leaflets and education must be provided (Marsden 2007). In entropion cases, the older patient must be taught how to perform lid taping and how often to do it. Patient empowerment is essential to promote patient-centred care and self-caring.

- The importance of maintaining good hygiene principles must be strongly emphasised when cleaning the lids and instilling eye medications (Watkinson & Seewoodhary 2008b).

- Pre-operative and post-operative care must be given at the correct time and the patient's and carer's understanding must be carefully evaluated (Marsden 2007).

- Effective therapeutic communication is essential in order to involve the patient as much as possible in their own care (Smith & Field 2011). If the older patient is from an ethnic group, the ophthalmic nurse has a duty of care to provide reassurance and information that is clearly understood (Smith & Field 2011) to help reassure the patient and carer.

- Maintaining eye contact and active listening are the basis for effective communication.

- Accurate record-keeping is essential when planning patient care. Confidentiality, patient dignity and respect must always be maintained (NMC 2008, NMC 2009a).

Blepharitis

Blepharitis is an inflammatory condition of the eyelids that can occur in patients of any age, from children to older people (Din & Patel 2012). The eyelid margins are lined with a series of oil glands that normally produce a thin, clear, oily material. This is essential for the stability of the tear film, as well as for protecting the skin of the eyelid from chronic exposure to the wet tears. Some of the glands are associated with the lashes and a second set of glands directly behind the lashes, called meibomian glands, produce meibum, which is essential in preserving the normal tear film on the ocular surface. Patients with blepharitis have unexplained inflammation of these glands. Figure 6.12 (see page 120) shows a severe blepharitis with corneal involvement.

Din & Patel (2012) state that the National Health Service reported that blepharitis accounted for 5% of all eye disorders in the UK.

The pathophysiology of blepharitis

The pathophysiology of blepharitis is a rather complex multifactorial process, which includes abnormal lid margin secretions, microbial involvement and a dysfunctional tear film (Jackson 2008). Changes in the quantity and quality of the lid margin secretions, alongside invasion by pathogens (Din & Patel 2012), result in instability and thinning of the tear film. This leads to rapid tear evaporation, increased tear osmolarity and inflammatory cytokine production, which precipitate the symptoms of blepharitis (Bowling 2011).

Din & Patel (2012) recommend that blepharitis should be classified as either anterior or posterior, each of which has its own pathophysiological process. The anterior type affects the anterior portion of the lid margin. There are three mechanisms involved:

1. Direct bacterial lid infection

2. Reaction to the endotoxins or exotoxins produced by the bacteria

3. Cell-mediated delayed hypersensitivity reaction to antigens.

These pathogens may include Staphylococcus epidermis, Staphylococcus aureus and Propionibacterium acnes (Lindstrom et al. 2010). Enzymes released by the pathogens cause scaling, crusting, redness of lid margin, with chronic states leading to ulcerative blepharitis. This eventually causes the lashes to drop out – a condition known as madarosis. Trichiasis, punctuate keratopathy and marginal keratitis may also occur. Trichiasis means ingrowing eyelashes, which tend to scratch the cornea, resulting in corneal abrasion and corneal ulceration (Kanski 2007). The toxin released by the bacteria damages the cornea, causing punctate keratopathy. The toxin can also result in type 4 hypersensitivity reaction, thus leading to the formation of marginal keratitis (see Figure 6.12).

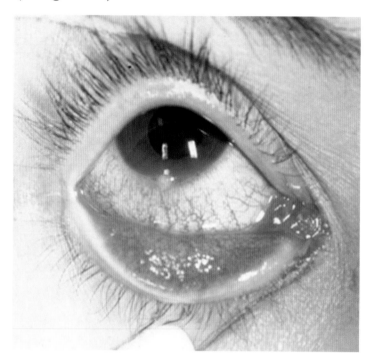

Figure 6.12: Blepharitis with corneal complication – marginal keratitis
Source: From UWL Media Services 2013

Posterior blepharitis is strongly associated with meibomian gland disease, with changes in the architecture of the gland openings (Din & Patel 2012). The symptoms also include distortion of meibum constituents and inflammatory lid changes. The oily secretion becomes thick and the flow gets blocked. A chalazion may result (Kanski 2007).

The lipid profile in meibomian gland secretion can be altered by age, menopause, androgen deficiency, bacteria, and autoimmune disease such as Sjogren's syndrome (Din & Patel 2012). A high ratio of omega-6 to omega-3 has been implicated in the state of inflammation and meibomian gland secretion. This thickened meibum can result in reduced delivery of meibum to the ocular surface and an obstructive meibomian gland state, leading to an unstable tear film and dry eyes. The cause is often unknown (Din & Patel 2012). The condition waxes and wanes, with periods when the eyes are comfortable. Older people often complain of a burning, itchy and sore feeling in their eyes, which is worse on waking up.

Managing older patients with blepharitis

A rigorous approach to eyelid hygiene is essential, and this regime should be continued even after the condition has apparently cleared. Older patients should be instructed to wash their face at least twice daily and hair should be kept clean and free of dandruff, as should eyebrows (Stollery *et al.* 2010).

There is no treatment for blepharitis because the disorder cannot be eradicated but only managed so that the patient obtains relief from the symptoms (Kanski & Bowling 2011). There are four steps involved in managing blepharitis (Kanski 2007), beginning with good lid hygiene.

Step 1

The first step involves placing a face cloth under warm water, then holding it against the closed eyelids for 2 minutes. The warmth of the cloth raises the temperature of the eyelids and takes the oils above their melting point. This results in thinning and greater flow of the oils. It softens the material that is on the eyelid margins and helps decompress those glands that may be blocked by excessive oil.

The eyelid should be gently wiped with a cotton bud to remove the excessive oil. Any crustiness will also be removed by the cotton bud. It is important that the patient carries out this routine daily, preferably in the morning. This should be seen as a process no different from washing their face or brushing their teeth every morning. It is important to inform older people that the accumulated oily material is a good breeding ground for bacteria, which can cause conjunctivitis and eye irritation.

Step 2

This involves applying topical antibiotic to the base of the lashes before bedtime, and this treatment is sufficient to bring the condition under control. Older people who have already developed secondary conjunctivitis will require a 10 to 14-day course of a topical antibiotic. Systemic antibiotics are rarely needed, except when topical preparations fail to work or secondary infections of the meibomian glands occur (Din & Patel 2012).

Step 3

This step is for those patients who have significant thickening of the secretions from the meibomian glands or a history of recurrent chalazions complicating their blepharitis. These patients are prescribed a systemic antibiotic, such as Tetracycline 250 mg, taken once-daily for three months, and this is often extended up to six months (Whittpenn 1995). Patients with ocular rosacea and meibomian gland disease, who are unresponsive to eyelid hygiene, respond well to oral Tetracyclines (Jackson 2008).

Step 4

This is the final step for older patients with severe active inflammatory changes on their lid margins, who are in extreme discomfort. Symptoms often settle down with the use of a combined antibiotic steroid ointment massaged on the eyelid margins (Pavan-Langston 2007). Patients must be regularly reviewed as steroid can result in cataracts or glaucoma. Use of artificial tears can help improve tear function and reduce inflammation (Din & Patel 2012).

Essential fatty acids can play a major role in the treatment of blepharitis and dry eyes (Sawant & Manoj 2006). They act by decreasing inflammation and cell apoptosis and improving the polar profiles of the meibomian gland secretion, thus increasing the oil and water layers of the tear film. These essential fatty acids include omega-3 EFA and omega-6 EFA. Sources of omega-3 EFA include coldwater fish, soya, flaxseeds and fenugreek seeds. Sources of omega-6 EFA are almonds, eggs, wholegrains, raw nuts, legumes and groundnut oil. Older people should be encouraged to incorporate these foods in their diet.

Practical nursing considerations

- Inform older people about the benefits of carrying out lid hygiene daily (Din & Patel 2012).
- Advise older patients to keep sufficient supplies of cotton buds and to use sterile water for lid cleaning.
- Provide information leaflets and read them aloud with the patient or carer to promote concordance (Watkinson & Seewoodhary 2007).
- Reassure patients that they are not 'dirty' and remind them that they are in control of their own care. It is dignifying for older people to know that this is a common eye disorder (NMC 2008).
- Advise them to eat a healthy diet and adopt a healthy lifestyle.
- They should not share towels with others.
- They must use medications as prescribed (Watkinson & Seewoodhary 2007) and keep all medications in a safe place.
- They need to wash their hands before and after carrying out lid hygiene.
- They should visit the optometrist yearly.

Conclusion

In conclusion, external eye diseases in older patients must never be dismissed as trivial. A correct diagnosis is required, and appropriate care and treatment must be given. Older people with low immunity are more prone to developing sight-threatening complications.

The role of the healthcare practitioner is essential in patient empowerment. Maintaining effective therapeutic communication will ensure that older people get the care they deserve. Dry eye, entropion, ectropion and blepharitis are very common eye problems in older people. Growing old with good vision and comfortable eyes will ensure that older people can enjoy their retirement and social life. A holistic approach must be adopted for each patient.

In the next chapter, the challenges of managing older people with herpes zoster ophthalmicus will be explored and the role of healthcare professionals addressed.

References

Din, N. & Patel, N.N. (2012). Blepharitis – a review of diagnosis and management. *International Journal of Ophthalmic Practice*. **3** (4), 150–54.

Dry Eye Workshop Report (2007). A Mission Completed. *Ocular Surface*. **5** (2), 65–204.

Henderson W.J., (2013). Dry-eye management. *Optometry in Practice* **14**, (4) 137–146.

Jackson, W.B. (2008). Blepharitis: current strategies for diagnosis and management. *Canadian Journal of Ophthalmology*. **43**, 170–79.

Kanski, J. (2007). *Clinical Ophthalmology*. Oxford: Blackwell Publishing.

Kanski, J. & Bowling, B. (2011). *Clinical Ophthalmology: A Systematic Approach*. 7th edn. London: Elsevier.

Lam, H., Bleiden, L., de Paiva, C.S., Farley, W., Stern, M.E. & Pflugfelder, S.C. (2009). Tear cytokine profiles in dysfunctional tear syndrome. *American Journal of Ophthalmology*. **147** (2), 198–205.

Lindstrom, R., Donnenfeld, E.D. & Fouks, G.N. (2010). 'Blepharitis – update on research and management 2010' in *The New York Eye and Ear Infirmary, MedEcus, Ophthalmology Times – a Continuing Medical Education monograph*.

Marsden, J. (2002). Ophthalmic trauma in the emergency department. *Accident and Emergency Nursing*. **10** (3), 136–42.

Marsden, J. (2006). *Ophthalmic Care*. Chichester: Wiley-Blackwell.

Marsden, J. (2007). *An Evidence Base for Ophthalmic Nursing Practice*. Chichester: Wiley-Blackwell.

Moorfields Eye Hospital (2006). *Pharmacists Handbook*. London: Moorfields Eye Hospital, NHS Foundation Trust.

Nursing and Midwifery Council (2008). *The Code: Standards of Conduct, Performance and Ethics for Nurses*. London: NMC.

Nursing and Midwifery Council (2009a). *Record keeping: Guidance for Nurses and Midwives*. London: NMC.

Nursing and Midwifery Council (2009b). *Guidance for the care of older people*. London: NMC.

Pavan-Langston, D. (2008). *Manual of Ocular Diagnosis and Therapy*. Philadelphia PA, USA: Williams and Wilkins.

Riordan-Eva, P. & Whitcher, J.P. (2008). *Vaughan and Asbury's General Ophthalmology*. 17th edn. New York, NY, USA: Lange Medical Books/McGraw-Hill.

Royal National Institute of Blind People (2012). *NB The eye health and sight loss magazine for professionals*. 77, 4.

Royal National Institute of Blind People (2012). Under 'Research and policy', 'Older people and sight loss'. www.rnib.org.uk/services-we-offer-advice-professionals-social-care-professionals/working-older-people (Last accessed: 7 May 2014).

Sawant, M. & Manoj, B. (Feb/Mar 2006). Role of essential fatty acids in the management of blepharitis and dry eye. *Eye News*. 9–12 www.pinpoint-scotland.com/ (Last accessed 8 May 2014).

Schaumberg, D.A. (2011). 'Physicians' understanding of dry eye disease' in *EUROTIMES supplement,* 10.

Schaumberg, D.A., Dana, R., Buring, J.E. & Sullivan, D.A. (2009). Prevalence of dry eye disease among US men; estimates from the Physicians' Health Studies. *Archives of Ophthalmology.* **127** (6), 763–68.

Seewoodhary, R. & Watkinson, S. (2009). Eye care in older people. *Nursing Standard.* **23** (35), 48–56.

Smith, J.A. (2007). The epidemiology of dry eye disease; report of the Epidemiology Subcommittee of the International Dry Eye Workshop. *Ocular Surface.* **5** (2), 93–107.

Smith, B. & Field, L. (2011). *An essential guide for nurses and healthcare workers in primary and secondary care.* Essex: Pearson Education.

Standing, M. (2011). *Clinical Judgement and Decision Making for Nursing Students.* Exeter: Learning Matters Ltd.

Stollery, R., Shaw, M. & Lee, M. (2010). *Ophthalmic Nursing.* 3rd edn. Oxford: Wiley-Blackwell.

Tornquist, A.L. (2012). Dry eye disease: simple to diagnose but complex to manage. *International Journal of Ophthalmic Practice.* **3** (5), 194–202.

Vafidis, G. (2007). 'Loss of vision'. www.gponline.com/Clinical/article/942686/Clinical-Review---Loss-vision/ (Last accessed: 1 April 2014).

Watkinson, S. & Seewoodhary, R. (2007). Common conditions and practical considerations in eye care. *Nursing Standard.* **21** (44), 42–47.

Watkinson, S. & Seewoodhary, R. (2008a). Ocular complications associated with diabetes mellitus. *Nursing Standard.* **22** (27), 51–57.

Watkinson, S. & Seewoodhary, R. (2008b). Administering eye medications. *Nursing Standard.* **22** (18), 42–48

Whittpenn, J.R. (1995). Eye scrub: Simplifying the management of blepharitis. *Journal of Ophthalmic Nursing & Technology.* **14** (1), 25–28.

Chapter 7

The older person with herpes zoster ophthalmicus

Susan Watkinson

This chapter covers

- Introduction
- Herpes zoster ophthalmicus – an overview
- Pathophysiology
- Risk factors
- Clinical features
- Complications
- Diagnosing herpes zoster ophthalmicus
- Current approaches to treatment
- Clinical management and the health and social care professional's role
- Future perspectives
- Conclusion

Introduction

This chapter will focus on the role of the health and social care professional in the clinical management of older people with herpes zoster ophthalmicus. Initially an overview of the condition and its associated pathophysiology will be presented. This will be followed by an examination of the risk factors, clinical features, diagnosis, approaches to treatment, the main complications (including post-herpetic neuralgia and ocular complications), and preventative measures. Current debates and future perspectives on the management of this condition will also be considered. Emphasis will be placed on the importance of providing the care required to support older patients during their treatment and subsequent rehabilitation from this debilitating viral disease.

Herpes zoster ophthalmicus – an overview

Herpes zoster (also known as shingles) is a common neurocutaneous infection caused by the human herpes virus type 3, the same virus that is responsible for chickenpox (Wiafe 2003). When the eye is involved, the virus is referred to as herpes zoster ophthalmicus.

Herpes zoster, characterised by a painful skin rash with blisters, is common in older people and immune-compromised and debilitated patients (Kang et al. 2009). One-fifth of the population, mainly older people, will present with herpes zoster during their lifetime (Opstelten & Zaal 2005). The incidence of herpes zoster ophthalmicus ranges from 2.2 per 1000 to 3.4 per 1000 people per year. In older patients, the incidence is approximately 10 people per 1000 annually. One in every 100 individuals will develop the condition during their lifetime (Opstelten & Zaal 2005). Many health and social care professionals are likely to encounter older patients with herpes zoster ophthalmicus, and these professionals have an important role to play in the care and management of people with this debilitating condition.

Economic impact on health services

Herpes zoster represents a significant healthcare burden among older people, even in those who are healthy (Chua & Chen 2010). Gauthier et al. (2009) examined management costs in immuno-competent patients with herpes zoster and found that the mean direct cost was £103 per patient. The costs of treating patients with post-herpetic neuralgia after diagnosis were £341 per episode after one month and £397 per episode after three months respectively. Gauthier et al. (2009) also confirmed that herpes zoster and post-herpetic neuralgia costs increased markedly with pain severity. In patients under the age of 65 years, acute herpes zoster is estimated to cost £526 per episode, when the costs to wider society resulting from loss of productivity are included (Wareham & Breuer 2007). The indirect costs, of reduced quality of life as a result of pain and disability, are impossible to calculate but nevertheless significant (Chua & Chen 2010).

Pathophysiology

The primary chickenpox (varicella) infection is believed to originate after exposure to infectious respiratory droplets and their subsequent entry through direct contact with an infected mucosal surface, such as the conjunctiva (Chua & Chen 2010). The most appropriate method of infection control during the primary varicella zoster virus (VZV) infection is respiratory isolation. The VZV quickly replicates in mononuclear cells of regional lymph nodes, and viraemia – where viruses enter the bloodstream – occurs within four to six days, resulting in systemic dissemination of the virus. Further replication occurs in the visceral organs and a secondary viraemia, leading to a generalised highly pruritic vesicular skin rash, which typically occurs 10–21 days after the initial exposure (Chua & Chen 2010).

During the primary infection, some viruses enter the sensory nerve endings in the skin and then proceed up the sensory nerve axon to the neuronal cell body at the dorsal root and cranial sensory (trigeminal) ganglia. Within the nuclei of these nerve cells, VZV may remain dormant for many years, even throughout a lifespan. However, it is the reactivation of this virus that usually results in a vesicular skin eruption, localised to one, two or three dermatomes (areas of skin that are mainly supplied by a single nerve). Reactivation of the VZV is related to diminished cell-mediated immunity (Chua & Chen 2010). Herpes zoster ophthalmicus occurs when the dormant VZV in the trigeminal ganglion, which involves the ophthalmic division of the fifth cranial nerve, becomes reactivated (Vallejo-Garcia et al. 2009).

Acute herpes zoster usually involves one nerve root on one side of the body, and this explains why herpes zoster always occurs on one side of the face (Johnson 2003). Once reactivated, the virus travels along the nerve fibres of the ophthalmic division of the sensory trigeminal nerve to cause the classic features of the condition (Catron & Hern 2008). Figure 7.1 (page 128) presents these classic features. Normally, the eyes and surrounding tissues are connected to sensory nerves that have physiological protective functions. For example, the cornea is a structure that is normally protected against trauma, dryness, exposure and infection, but it will become desensitised by the VZV, making it prone to such complications (Catron & Hern 2008).

Risk factors

The risk factors for developing herpes zoster include:

- Ageing
- Cancer
- Chemotherapy
- Emotional stress
- Fatigue
- Physical stress from illness
- Poor nutrition
- Radiation therapy
- Systemic disorders that weaken the immune system.

(Wareham & Breuer 2007)

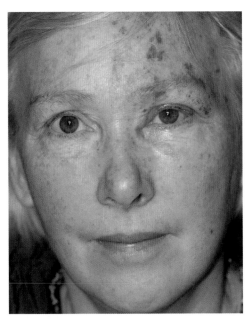

Figure 7.1: The classic features of herpes zoster ophthalmicus

Clinical features

Older patients with herpes zoster ophthalmicus can present with both extra-ocular as well as more specific ocular features. The two sets of features can sometimes occur simultaneously (Wiafe 2003).

Extra-ocular features include:

- Malaise, pain, itching, photophobia, and low-grade fever up to a week before a skin rash appears.
- The rash usually commences with progressive pain sensations, accompanied by hypersensitive areas on the forehead.
- Erythematous macules (spots or stained areas) appear and progress to form clusters of papules (pimples) and clear vesicles (small collections of fluid in the epidermis) in the affected dermatome.
- New skin lesions usually continue to appear for three to five days.
- The rash progresses through stages of pustulation and crusting.
- A rash in the dermatome of the nasociliary nerve (Hutchinson's sign) may indicate ophthalmic complications.

(Opstelten & Zaal 2005)

A wide range of symptoms affecting the eye may occur during the various phases of herpes zoster ophthalmicus. These include:

- Peri-orbital oedema in the early phase.
- Severe skin inflammation may produce late-phase contraction scars, leading to incomplete eyelid closure and corneal exposure.
- Conjunctivitis
- Episcleritis – localised inflammation of the thin layer of vascularised connective tissue overlying the sclera.
- Scleritis – a primary inflammation of the sclera often associated with an underlying systemic infection or autoimmune disease.
- Keratitis – inflammation of the cornea.
- Reduced corneal sensitivity.
- Mild uveitis – inflammation of one or all sections of the uveal tract, which comprises the iris, ciliary body and choroid, with temporary elevated intra-ocular pressure.

(Opstelten & Zaal 2005)

Complications

The two main complications of herpes zoster ophthalmicus are post-herpetic neuralgia (PHN) and ocular involvement (Vallejo-Garcia et al. 2009). Ocular infection occurs when the ophthalmic division of the trigeminal nerve is involved.

Other complications may include:

- Conjunctivitis
- Keratitis, iridocyclitis
- Choroiditis
- Papillitis (inflammation of the intra-ocular optic nerve)
- Oculomotor nerve palsy (lesions of the third cranial nerve, affecting the extra-ocular muscles and limiting eye movements)
- Retinitis
- Optic atrophy (a non-specific response to optic nerve damage from any cause)
- Dry eyes and lid scarring.

(Wareham & Breuer 2007)

Post-herpetic neuralgia

PHN is partly the result of neuronal loss and subsequent scar formation in that part of the sensory ganglion and dorsal horn of the spinal cord damaged by the reactivation of the virus (Chua and Chen, 2010). They further suggest that the neuropathic disease experienced by the individual is also very heterogeneous resulting from complex mechanisms of action as yet incompletely understood (Chua and Chen, 2010).

PHN is described as neuropathic pain that persists or develops after the dermatomal rash has healed (Vallejo-Garcia et al. 2009). The indicators for PHN are older age, severe acute pain and rash, shorter duration of rash before consultation (this suggests the trigeminal nerves are severely inflamed), and ocular involvement. It occurs in 36.6% of patients over the age of 60 years and in 47.5% of patients over the age of 70 years with herpes zoster ophthalmicus (Vallejo-Garcia et al. 2009).

The clinical spectrum of PHN is wide-ranging. It can present as mild discomfort lasting for a few months to a severe debilitating pain, which may persist throughout a patient's lifetime. Sometimes the pain is severe enough to disrupt a person's sleep, work and activities of daily living.

The condition is very difficult to treat once established, making the prevention of herpes zoster a key healthcare target (Chua & Chen 2010). Indeed, Vallejo-Garcia et al. (2009) report that persistent PHN has been linked to suicide in patients over the age of 70 years.

Diagnosing herpes zoster ophthalmicus

Diagnosis of herpes zoster ophthalmicus is made by a combination of history-taking and physical examination (Catron & Hern 2008). Physical examination consists of an ophthalmic assessment. This should involve external examination of the eye, assessment of visual fields and acuity, extra-ocular movements and pupillary response, fundoscopy, intra-ocular measurement, anterior chamber slit lamp examination and corneal examination, with and without staining (Catron & Hern 2008).

Viral culture and molecular techniques are available when a definitive diagnosis is required (Vallejo-Garcia et al. 2009).

Overall, prompt referral to an ophthalmologist is indicated when the ophthalmic division of the trigeminal nerve and nasociliary nerve are involved (Hutchinson's sign) and when there is unexplained ocular redness with pain, or complaints of visual problems (Vallejo-Garcia et al. 2009). The diagnosis of herpes zoster is usually based on clinical observation of the characteristic rash.

Current approaches to treatment

A key approach involves the use of systemic oral anti-viral agents, which reduce both the acute pain of herpes zoster and the incidence of PHN. Aciclovir, for example, if administered within 72 hours of the onset of the rash, has been shown to be effective in several ways. It can reduce the percentage of eye disorders in patients with herpes zoster ophthalmicus from 50% to 20–30%, alleviate acute pain, and prevent or limit the duration or severity of post-herpetic neuralgia (Vallejo-Garcia et al. 2009).

In clinical practice, however, the second-generation antiviral drugs, such as famciclovir and valaciclovir, although more costly, may be more effective than aciclovir because only three, rather than five, daily doses are required and patients are therefore more likely to adhere to the treatment regimen (Opstelten & Zaal 2005).

Another approach is to use corticosteroids, tricyclic anti-depressants, and gabapentin and opioids, which also reduce acute pain and may help reduce PHN (Wareham & Breuer 2007). Tricyclic anti-depressants, gabapentin, opioids and lidocaine patches are also effective in treating established post-herpetic neuralgia (Wareham & Breuer 2007).

Quan et al. (2007) point out that in clinical practice, many PHN sufferers are refractory to available therapy. Thus, patient satisfaction, especially among older patients, is further compromised by intolerable side-effects such as confusion, dizziness, sedation, nausea or other gastrointestinal disturbances. Therefore understanding of the disease is crucial in being able to direct treatment towards dealing with the underlying mechanisms of pain.

Herpes zoster ophthalmicus and post-herpetic neuralgia

Oral opioids and non-steroidal anti-inflammatory drugs are frequently indicated to relieve pain and promote comfort in patients with PHN resulting from herpes zoster ophthalmicus. Their effects may be enhanced by the use of cycloplegic eye drops in patients showing signs of iritis, such as pain, photophobia and blurred vision.

The cycloplegic eye drops relax the ciliary muscles, paralysing accommodation, thereby relieving spasm and ocular pain, and relaxing the eye. Accommodation refers to the way the eye adjusts to see things at near distances. This is achieved by changing the shape of the lens through the ciliary muscle, thus focusing a clear image on the retina. Cycloplegic (dilating) eye drops will paralyse the ciliary muscle, thus relaxing accommodation and preventing the lens from changing its shape to see near objects.

The overall effect is to increase patient comfort (Catron & Hern, 2008). In addition, eye ointment (such as a lubricant) may be prescribed to protect the cornea from dryness and nerve damage, and, again, to promote the patient's comfort (Shaw et al. 2010).

Clinical management and the health and social care professional's role

The health and social care professional's role in managing the care of older patients with herpes zoster ophthalmicus in the community will now be discussed. Most patients will be cared for at home. In this context, the key aspects of the healthcare professional's role include effective communication and counselling, management of pain and depression, promoting adherence to medication, ophthalmic and skin care management, and health promotion and education.

Communication and counselling

Good communication and counselling skills are pivotal to effective management. Older patients, in particular, may be frightened by the distressing nature of the condition and will require reassurance and support (Shaw et al. 2010). Some of the major fears involve the potential ocular complications that may occur, the possibility of sight loss and acquiring poor body image as a result of skin disfigurement (Shaw et al. 2010). Another anxiety relates to patient perceptions about being infectious and transmitting the infection to other people. It is therefore important to provide opportunities to talk to older patients about herpes zoster ophthalmicus and its treatment, and answer any queries they may have about this condition.

Making older patients aware of the side-effects of their medication is also crucial. Amitriptyline, for example, is associated with drowsiness, dry mouth and constipation (BNF 2010). Side-effects of the main anti-viral medications used, such as aciclovir, famiciclovir and valaciclovir, include nausea, vomiting, abdominal pain, diarrhoea, headache, fatigue, sensitive rash, and in some cases, renal insufficiency (BNF 2010).

It is particularly advisable to follow a healthy diet during the first week of treatment in order to help boost the immune system (Kanski & Bowling 2011). An adequate intake of fluids is equally important in preventing dehydration.

Older patients also need to be reassured that they will receive ongoing treatment in the outpatient department. The importance of attendance must be stressed, as they may develop a few complications such as dry eyes and corneal lesions, which could compromise their sight (Watkinson & Seewoodhary 2011).

Pain and depression

Patients with herpes zoster ophthalmicus will feel unwell because of the severe facial pain associated with the acute phase of the condition (Catron & Hern 2008, Vallejo-Garcia et al. 2009), or the later complication of persistent PHN. This may lead to depression (Ang et al.

2010). The facial pain can be exacerbated by the slightest touch, and the onset of depression may lead to loss of employment and social isolation (Wareham & Breuer 2007). Pain is a strong predictor of the onset and persistence of depression.

Furthermore, because depression lowers the patient's pain threshold, it is in turn a powerful predictor of pain, particularly persistent pain (Ang et al. 2010). Concurrent pain and depression have a much greater effect than either disorder alone on the patient's functional status and use of healthcare resources (Ang et al. 2010).

Quality of life

Clearly, the effects of pain and depression may compromise the patient's quality of life to a greater or lesser extent. To this end, some quantitative measures have been used to acknowledge these effects by measuring quality of life in patients with herpes zoster and PHN. One such measure is the Likert Scale, measuring pain on a 0 to 10 scale, where 0 equals no pain, and 10 equals severe pain (Quan et al. 2007).

The Zoster Brief Pain Inventory (ZBPI) can also be used. This is an assessment containing zoster-specific modifications, as opposed to the more general Brief Pain Inventory, which is a widely used questionnaire to evaluate pain. The ZBPI is designed to capture zoster pain severity and interference with functional status in seven spheres of daily life, including:

- General activity
- Mood
- Walking
- Work
- Relations with others
- Sleep
- Enjoyment of life.

Knowledge and use of such scales in practice results in more effective planning and care management of older patients in order to help reduce the effects of pain and depression on their daily lives.

Depending on the severity of the pain, an appropriate analgesic should be prescribed. Some patients may also require referral to a pain clinic. A tricyclic anti-depressant such as amitriptyline is usually prescribed to help manage pain-related depression. Doses normally start at 10–25mg at night and are increased gradually (BNF 2010). Some of the symptoms of depression likely to be encountered include altered mood, anger, anxiety, confused thinking, decreased self-esteem, fatigue, irritability and sleep disturbances (NICE 2009).

Again, the use of tricyclic anti-depressants may benefit some older patients who are experiencing sleep disturbances due to chronic pain, since one side-effect of these drugs is sedation. However, the overall benefits of these drugs may not be felt for three to four weeks (BNF 2010).

Undoubtedly, counselling skills remain important in helping and supporting older patients and their families to manage some of the consequences of pain-related depression (Watkinson & Seewoodhary 2011). Taking the time to listen actively to patients will enable them to deal with their emotions much better (Watkinson & Scott 2010). Likewise, exploring older people's fears, anxieties, misapprehensions and feelings of anger will allow them to allay some perceived problems. Healthcare professionals should always aim to provide a quiet environment and respect the older person's dignity when trying to promote effective communication within a therapeutic relationship (Watkinson & Scott 2010).

Adherence to treatment – the psychosocial role

Loss of self-esteem as a result of depression can make it difficult for older patients to stick to treatment regimes (Chia et al. 2006). Knowledge of psychosocial theory is useful to the health and social care professional when helping to manage the patient in this situation. Firstly, it is important to appreciate the effect of individual health belief systems on medication adherence, especially in older people (Chia et al. 2006).

Fundamentally, people considering a change in their behaviour engage in a cost-benefit or utility analysis (Becker 1974). This means that the decision to make a change will be influenced by an evaluation of its feasibility and its benefits weighed against its costs (Becker 1974). Older patients, for example, may not believe in the effectiveness of the medication they are taking and may feel that the side-effects outweigh the benefits. Conversely, if older patients perceive the prescribed medication as being beneficial or necessary, they are more likely to adhere to the treatment (Chia et al. 2006).

Self-esteem is a key component in motivation (Tones et al. 1990). How older people view themselves will have a major influence on their readiness to make positive decisions about their health (Tones et al. 1990). Clearly, loss of self-esteem will have adverse effects on positive decision-making. In this situation, it is vital to support the older person in increasing the incentive to change, discussing and reinforcing the implications of non-treatment for their condition, and importantly raising their level of self-efficacy so that they feel capable of carrying out and following the prescribed treatment (Bandura 1977).

Generally, adopting a positive attitude towards older patients and stressing the benefits of adherence to treatment will help increase their belief in the importance of maintaining control over their condition. It is equally important to listen carefully to what older patients want to say and allow them to talk about negative and difficult feelings related to their illness and treatment (Wilkes *et al.* 2003). This is pivotal to the maintenance of a therapeutic relationship.

Ophthalmic and skin care management

The older patient's skin must be kept clean and prescribed topical treatment should be applied to reduce the itching and discomfort. Community nurses should observe the skin rash regularly in order to assess any changes and monitor for signs of infection. Older patients may also require support and assistance from informal carers or family members (Watkinson & Seewoodhary 2011).

Eye care is important to promote patient comfort and to prevent the onset of infection. It involves good hygiene practice, daily eye dressings and keeping the eyelids clean by means of regular bathing. This can be undertaken by the informal carer initially, and later by the older patient to promote self-care. Eye medication should be administered as prescribed. The eyes must also be observed for any changes resulting from treatment (for example, pupillary dilation if mydriatic eye drops have been prescribed, since blurred vision will be experienced for a short time following instillation). Other observations include complications such as a corneal infection, which manifests as a red eye and a hazy cornea. The latter indicates that the integrity of the cornea is compromised and unable to maintain clarity (Riordan-Eva & Whitcher 2008).

Photophobia can be managed by ensuring that bright lighting is dimmed within the home environment. However, older patients' safety must be taken into account, and any obstacles likely to cause falls or injury should be removed. Patients should also be encouraged to wear dark glasses when going outside (Watkinson & Seewoodhary 2011).

Body image

Loss of self-esteem may also result from disturbances to body image following facial skin disfigurement. The health and social care professional should encourage older patients to take an interest in their personal appearance. Again, effective communication skills are central to the sensitive management of any psychological issues associated with altered body image (Rumsey *et al.* 2002). The health and social care professional needs to demonstrate a positive interest in older patients by spending time listening and talking to them. Reassurance also needs to be provided about their external appearance. Non-verbal communication such as the skilful and appropriate use of touch and demonstrations of affection (for example, a handshake or a brief, gentle touch on the patient's arm) can convey a genuine sense of empathy and caring.

Health promotion and education

Health and social care professionals also need to raise public awareness about how to prevent herpes zoster. Knowledge and understanding of the current herpes zoster vaccine is essential so that healthy older patients aged 60 years or more can be provided with up-to-date information about the safety and effectiveness of this method of prevention. It is important to explain that vaccination is targeted at those aged 60 years or older because of the decline in the immune system that occurs with the ageing process. Some markers of T-cell immunity are known to be enhanced following vaccination.

The herpes zoster vaccine can significantly reduce the burden of herpes zoster among older people and its introduction has been demonstrated to be cost-effective (Chua & Chen 2010). It is similar to the paediatric varicella zoster vaccine, but of higher potency. It contains approximately 14 times more virus than the paediatric vaccine. However, some problems do exist with the herpes zoster vaccine as it is composed of a live attenuated virus, which signals important contraindications for its use (see below). These contraindications limit the protection offered by the vaccine, especially among the highest-risk groups in the population (Chen & Chua 2010). They include:

- Anaphylactic reactions to any component of the vaccine
- Pregnancy
- Primary or acquired immunodeficiencies such as haematological malignancy, human immunodeficiency virus with acquired immunodeficiency syndrome, recent haematopoietic stem cell transplantation and patients receiving immunosuppressive therapy.

Future perspectives

The key issue is that there are gaps in medical knowledge related to the use of the herpes zoster vaccine that need to be addressed. Filling these gaps will require ongoing research. In the UK, a vaccine is currently available for 'at risk' groups (including patients with chronic medical conditions such as chronic renal failure, diabetes mellitus, rheumatoid arthritis, chronic pulmonary disease) and for those who are not immune and work in an environment where they may become infected, such as health and social care professionals working in a hospital environment or community setting.

Conclusion

In summary, this chapter has discussed the role of the health and social care professional in managing the care of older people with herpes zoster ophthalmicus.

Initially it provided an overview of the condition and associated pathophysiology. It then examined the risk factors, clinical features, diagnosis, current approaches to treatment, complications such as post-herpetic neuralgia, and the herpes zoster vaccine as a key preventative measure for this condition. Importantly, there was in-depth discussion of the care required to support older patients during their treatment and subsequent rehabilitation. Particular reference was made to managing the pain and depression arising from herpes zoster ophthalmicus and the importance of counselling. Furthermore, the use of effective communication and psychosocial skills was seen as a means to facilitate adherence to treatment and promote quality of life.

The issues of pain and depression arising from debilitating disease were also explored. Although the relationship between depression and visual loss is one that deserves more consideration, regrettably its importance may sometimes be underestimated in clinical practice. The next chapter in this book seeks to address some of the important issues influencing this relationship, with reference to key age-related ocular diseases.

References

Ang, D.C., Bair, M.J. & Damush, T.M. (2010). Predictors of pain outcomes in patients with chronic musculoskeletal pain co-morbid with depression: results from a randomised controlled trial. *Pain Medicine.* **11** (4), 482–91.

Bandura, A. (1977). *Social Learning Theory.* Englewood Cliffs, NJ, USA: Prentice Hall.

Becker, M.H. (Ed) (1974). *The Health Belief Model and Personal Health Behaviour.* Thorofare, NJ, USA: Slack.

British National Formulary (2010). *British National Formulary No. 59.* London: British Medical Association and the Royal Pharmaceutical Society of Great Britain.

Catron, T. & Hern, H.G. (2008). Herpes zoster ophthalmicus. *Western Journal of Emergency Medicine.* **9** (3), 174–76.

Chia, L.R., Schlenck, E. A. & Dunbar-Jacob, J. (2006). Effect of personal and cultural beliefs on medication adherence in the elderly. *Drugs and Ageing.* **23** (3), 191–202.

Chua, J.V. & Chen, W.H. (2010). Herpes zoster vaccine for the elderly: boosting immunity. *Ageing Health.* **6** (2), 169–76.

Gaulthier, A., Breuer, J., Carrington, D., Martin, M. & Remy, V. (2009). Epidemiology and cost of herpes zoster and post-herpetic neuralgia in the United Kingdom. *Epidemiology and Infection.* **137** (1), 38–47.

Johnson, L. (2003). Effective pain management of post-herpetic neuralgia. *Nursing Times.* **99** (10), 32–34.

Kang, J.H., Ho, J.D., Chen, Y.H. & Lin, H.C. (2009). Increased risk of stroke after a herpes zoster attack: a population-based follow-up study. *Stroke.* **40** (11), 3443–48.

Kanski, J. & Bowling, B. (2011). *Clinical Ophthalmology: A Systematic Approach.* 7th edn. London: Elsevier.

National Institute for Health and Clinical Excellence (2009). 'Depression in Adults with a Chronic Physical Health Problem: Treatment and Management'. www.nccmh.org.uk/downloads/DCHP/CG91NICEGuideline.pdf (Last accessed: 24 April 2014)

Opstelten, W. & Zaal, M.J. (2005). Managing ophthalmic herpes zoster in primary care. *British Medical Journal.* **331** (7509), 147–51.

Quan, D., Cohrs, R.J., Mahalingam, R. & Gilden, D.H. (2007). Prevention of shingles: safety and efficacy of live zoster vaccine. *Therapeutics and Clinical Risk Management.* **3** (4), 633–39.

Riordan-Eva, P. & Whitcher, J.P. (eds) (2008). *Vaughan and Asbury's General Ophthalmology.* 17th edn. New York, NY, USA: McGraw-Hill.

Rumsey, N., Clarke, A. & Musa, M. (2002). Altered body image: the psychosocial needs of patients. *British Journal of Community Nursing.* **7** (11), 563–66.

Shaw, M.E., Lee, A. & Stollery, R. (2010). *Ophthalmic Nursing.* 4th edn. Chichester: Wiley-Blackwell.

Tones, B.K., Tilford, S. & Keeley Robinson, Y. (1990). *Health Education: Effectiveness and Efficiency.* London: Chapman and Hall.

Vallejo-Garcia, J.L., Vano-Galvan, S., Rayward, O. & Moreno-Martin, P. (2009). Painful eye with a facial rash. *Cleveland Clinic Journal of Medicine.* **76** (7), 410–12.

Wareham, D.W. & Breuer, J. (2007). Herpes zoster. *British Medical Journal.* **334** (7605), 1211–15.

Watkinson, S. & Scott, E. (2010). Care of patients undergoing intra-vitreal therapy. *Nursing Standard.* **24** (25), 42–47.

Watkinson, S. & Seewoodhary, R. (2011). Managing the care of patients with herpes zoster ophthalmicus. *Nursing Standard.* **25** (39), 35–40.

Wiafe, B. (2003). Herpes zoster ophthalmicus in HIV/AIDS. *Community Eye Health.* **16** (47), 35–36.

Wilkes, L.M., O'Baugh, J., Luke, S. & George, C. (2003). Positive attitude in cancer: patient perspectives. *Oncology Nursing Forum.* **30** (3), 412–16.

Chapter 8

Managing depression in visually impaired older people

Susan Watkinson

This chapter covers

- Introduction
- Defining depression
- Current approaches to treatment
- Clinical management and the health and social care professional's role
- The impact of sight loss and depression with reference to specific ocular diseases
- Future perspectives
- Conclusion

Introduction

This chapter focuses on the management of depression in older people with visual impairment. After a brief introduction to ageing, visual impairment and depression, a literature review will be presented in order to highlight significant studies from the existing evidence base and provide further background. The concept of depression will be defined, the main classifications outlined, and the signs and symptoms presented.

Current approaches to treatment will then be discussed, before examining the role of the health and social care professional in the clinical management of depression in older people with visual impairment. The impact of depression (following sight loss) on the quality of life of older people will be discussed at length, with reference to specific ocular diseases such as cataract, age-related macular degeneration (AMD) and chronic open-angle glaucoma (COAG). Future perspectives on the management of this clinical problem will finally be offered, before drawing some overall conclusions.

Ageing, visual impairment and depression

Older age is associated with decreased physical competence and increased prevalence of chronic illness (Hayman et al. 2007). Visual impairment is an important example of chronic illness and a cause of disability, which has a direct effect on physical function and performance (Hayman et al. 2007). By the age of 70, 9% of people have moderate or more severe visual loss, and this increases to 30% for people over 80 (Hayman et al. 2007).

Visually impaired older people are more likely to experience problems associated with functioning, which leads to depression (Evans et al. 2007). Furthermore, they have a noticeably higher rate of depression than sighted older people (Evans et al. 2007). Consequently, quality of life, general functioning, visual functioning and the ability to benefit from a range of rehabilitation approaches are all affected (Smith 2009). Cataract, AMD, COAG and diabetic retinopathy are all important examples of ocular conditions that can often lead to loss of sight-related quality of life and subsequent depression.

The link between depression and visual impairment

The following research evidence highlights a significant link between depression and visual disability. Hayman et al. (2007) investigated the associations between physical and visual disability and depression in a sample of 391 people, aged 75 and over, with a visual acuity of less than 6/24 (20/80). The results demonstrated that depression was common in this group, and impaired visual and physical functions were associated with the symptoms of depression.

Patients with AMD often express feelings of depression and thoughts of suicide (Lewis & Southwell 2006). Blyth (2006) confirmed this finding and also concluded that AMD patients were twice as likely to experience clinical depression, compared with people with normal vision. Brody et al. (2001) collected cross-sectional baseline data from a randomised controlled trial which found that, of 151 patients (mean age 80) with advanced AMD who had undergone formal diagnostic assessment, 49 (32.5%) had depressive disorder. This was twice the usual rate in older people.

Depression was strongly associated with vision-specific and general disability scores (Brody et al., 2001). Rovner et al.'s (2002) follow-up study of 51 AMD patients with recent loss of vision in the second eye assessed patients at baseline and six months later. Results showed that 17 (33%) had depression at baseline, with poorer visual acuity, greater visual disability and greater general disability. At six months' follow-up, those whose depression had worsened also had worsening visual and general function – independent of any change in visual acuity.

Evans *et al.* (2007) undertook a population-based cross-sectional study of 13,900 people aged 75 and older and found that 1,876 (13.5%) visually impaired people had a score of 6 or more on the Geriatric Depression Scale, compared with 639 (4.6%) people with good vision. However, no association was found between visual impairment and anxiety. Interestingly, Mabuchi *et al.* (2008), using the Hospital Anxiety and Depression Scale, found a high prevalence of both anxiety and depression in patients with COAG, a disorder characterised by loss of optic nerve fibres as a result of increased intra-ocular pressure.

The relationship between depression and diabetic retinopathy was discussed earlier, in Chapter 5 of this book, with reference to the longitudinal study carried out by Roy *et al.* (2007). This team administered the Beck Depression inventory to examine data about depression in relation to glycaemic control as a risk factor for diabetic retinopathy. They found that depression was significantly associated with poor glycaemic control and higher six-year progression to proliferative diabetic retinopathy in African-Americans with type 1 diabetes (Roy *et al.* 2007).

Defining depression

Depression refers to a wide range of mental health problems characterised by the absence of a positive affect, signalling a loss of interest and enjoyment in ordinary things and experiences, low mood, and a range of associated emotional, cognitive, physical and behavioural symptoms (NICE 2009a).

Depression may be categorised as mild, moderate or severe, based on a set of core and associate symptoms (Table 8.1, page 142). Core symptoms include persistent sadness, anhedonia (loss of pleasure) and fatigue. Associate symptoms include sleep and appetite disturbance, poor concentration, agitation, decreased libido, low self-confidence, suicidal thoughts and/or acts, and guilt (WHO 2011). These problems can become chronic or recurrent and may substantially impair an individual's ability to take care of their everyday responsibilities.

Depression in older people is often under-diagnosed and under-treated (SCIE 2006). This is particularly true of older people in residential and nursing homes and older people in the community (SCIE 2006). Older people also tend not to complain about being depressed and are more likely to refer to their physical symptoms.

Overall, depression causes great mental distress, and in a worst-case scenario can lead to suicide, which results in the loss of about 850,000 lives every year (WHO 2011).

Table 8.1: Categorising depression

Category of depression	Number of symptoms present	Core symptoms	Associate symptoms
Mild	Four	Persistent sadness, anhedonia, fatigue	Suicidal thoughts/acts
Moderate	Five to six	Persistent sadness, anhedonia, fatigue	Poor concentration, sleep disturbance, suicidal thoughts/acts
Severe	Seven or more	Persistent sadness, anhedonia, fatigue	Sleep disturbance, appetite disturbance, poor concentration, agitation, decreased libido, low self-confidence, suicidal thoughts/acts, guilt

(Adapted from National Institute for Health and Clinical Excellence 2009a)

Current approaches to treatment

Current approaches to treatment include psychosocial interventions (see Table 8.2, page 143) such as cognitive behavioural therapy (CBT), counselling and interpersonal therapy (IPT), as well as anti-depressant medication.

CBT, counselling and IPT, also known as talking therapies, can help people work out how to deal with negative thoughts and feelings, and make positive changes (Mental Health Foundation 2011). Currently, the Department of Health values such therapies. Its aim is to complete the nationwide Improving Access to Psychological Therapies programme and provide services for adults of all ages who have depression or anxiety disorders, paying particular attention to ensuring appropriate access for people over the age of 65 (DH 2011).

Mild to moderate depression

People with sub-threshold depressive symptoms or mild to moderate depression will initially receive appropriate low-intensity psychosocial interventions. People with persistent sub-threshold depressive symptoms or mild to moderate depression, who have not benefited from low-intensity psychosocial interventions, will then be offered anti-depressants or high-intensity interventions (NICE 2009a).

The side-effects of most anti-depressants are usually mild and tend to wear off after a couple of weeks (Royal College of Psychiatrists 2011). The newer anti-depressants, known as selective serotonin reuptake inhibitors (SSRIs), may make people feel nauseous initially and more anxious for a short time. The older anti-depressants can cause a dry mouth and constipation (Royal College of Psychiatrists 2011). Treatment can commence with an SSRI prescribed at a low dose, which can then be increased weekly to the maximum tolerated level for a sustained trial of at least eight weeks. If there has been no response at all after four weeks, a change in medication is indicated. Potential drug interactions, possible side-effects and drug costs all need to be carefully considered (NICE 2009a).

Moderate to severe depression

People with moderate to severe depression will receive a combination of anti-depressant medication and a high-intensity psychosocial intervention. People with severe depression receive a combination of anti-depressant therapy and individual CBT (NICE 2009a).

Table 8.2: Psychosocial interventions for depression

Cognitive behavioural therapy (CBT)	CBT is based on a cognitive model of emotional disorders, which proposes that an individual's mood and behaviour are determined by the way they perceive the world. Their world view depends on cognitions based on underlying assumptions and core beliefs derived from previous experiences (Beck *et al.* 1979).
Interpersonal therapy (IPT)	IPT focuses on current relationships and interpersonal interactions (NICE 2009a).
Counselling	Counselling denotes a professional relationship between a trained counsellor and an individual. Overall, it aims to provide an opportunity for a client to work towards living in a way they experience as more satisfying (DH 2000).

Clinical management and the health and social care professional's role

In primary care, older people with depression are managed by GPs and practice nurses. In this chapter, the focus is on managing depression in secondary care settings, such as hospitals, eye clinics and residential care homes.

In secondary care, the health and social care professional's role in managing depression in older people with visual impairment includes the effective delivery of psychosocial care to help alleviate the depression. This provides a basis for resuming independence and maintaining a quality of life. Recognising and assessing the symptoms of depression, providing psychosocial support for the older person and their family or caregivers, and imparting information and advice about formal counselling and emotional support services are all important aspects of care.

Recognising depression

The NICE (2011) quality standard on depression has 13 statements that define high-quality care. These include ensuring that people who may have depression receive an assessment that identifies the severity of symptoms, the degree of associated functional impairment and the duration of the episode. Thus, it is important for the health and social care professional to be alert to the symptoms of depression in older patients with visual impairment, particularly in those patients with a history of depression.

Two useful questions to ask in detecting depression are whether during the past month the older person has been bothered by feeling 'down', depressed or hopeless, and whether the person has been having little interest or pleasure in doing things. If the older person gives 'yes' responses, action may then be taken by the healthcare professionals to conduct further assessments using the Geriatric Assessment Scale and to assist with the Zung Self-Rating Depression Scale to support their judgement. After monitoring the course of the depression, the older person may need to be referred to the appropriate healthcare professional for help and treatment (NICE 2009a).

Psychosocial care

The prospect of sight loss can be very daunting and depressing for the older person so it is essential to develop a trusting and therapeutic relationship in order to explore their feelings and fears about blindness (Watkinson & Scott 2010). Effective use of counselling skills, active listening, and positive responses are all helpful. It is also vital for healthcare professionals to respect the older person's privacy and dignity because of the possible stigma and discrimination that can be associated with depression (NICE 2009a). Conducting consultations and interviews in a quiet environment can help maintain privacy and dignity.

It is important to adopt a positive attitude when supporting the older person, particularly when exploring treatment options, and to promote the message of eventual recovery (NICE 2009a). However, it is also true that some older people may feel a strong need to express their anger, fear and other negative emotions about their sight loss and treatment during conversations (Tod 2011). Such feelings should be acknowledged by the health and social care professional, and opportunities given to talk about them with the older person as part of a therapeutic process (Wilkes *et al.* 2003).

Information giving

Providing the older person with information about depression and its treatment is essential. Family or carers should also be involved in the information-exchange process to enhance their knowledge and understanding of vision-related depression and to enable them to give continuing support to the person. Information can be offered about counselling and emotional support services, self-help groups, patient support groups and other resources. Information can also be given about the Royal National Institute of Blind People (RNIB) telephone helpline, and in particular, the Macular Disease Society helpline for older people with AMD (Watkinson 2011). AMD International focuses on support through the sharing of personal accounts and experiences with other AMD patients who have depression.

For older patients with diabetic retinopathy, a counselling and psychological support service is available. The International Glaucoma Association also provides help and support. In addition, the older person can be provided with information about local GP access as part of the statutory services available. Some local charities also offer face-to-face counselling (Watkinson 2011).

The impact of sight loss and depression with reference to specific ocular diseases

Understanding the reasons for depression associated with sight loss is critical in trying to help the older person and their family to manage the situation. Family members, especially spouses, can often become depressed themselves when trying to cope with the person's anger, distress and frustration (Bambara *et al.* 2009). Self-sufficiency and self-esteem are diminished as the person mourns the loss of their ability to see. Again, the family often shares this sense of grief. Nevertheless, it is important to be honest and dispel false hopes that either medical or surgical interventions will improve existing vision (Bambara *et al.* 2009), with the exception of cataract surgery.

Cataract

In older people with cataracts, it is important to find out what their expectations of ageing are, and explore their health beliefs and attitudes about their gradual loss of sight, how the cataracts have contributed to this, and how it is affecting them. Many have the mistaken belief that sight is less important in older age and that the restrictive effect of vision loss should be accepted as part of growing old (Polack 2008). Cataract visual impairment can have a major negative effect on the quality of people's lives (Polack 2008). Depression can arise when people experience persistent difficulties with basic daily living activities such as cooking, reading, watching television or walking.

It is therefore important to offer explanation and reassure the older patient and their family that surgical removal of cataracts is effective in restoring a sighted quality of life. Restoring vision also reduces psychiatric and somatic symptoms (Unite for Sight 2011). In nursing home residents, Owsley et al. (2007) found significant improvements in vision-targeted health-related quality of life after cataract surgery.

Age-related macular degeneration

When older people with AMD discover there is no permanent cure for their eye condition, they may experience mental and emotional turmoil. This is particularly true for people with dry AMD, where there is a breakdown or thinning of the layer of retinal pigment epithelial cells in the macula, and for which there is no treatment. Regular monitoring and support will be required, however, and the use of low vision aids can help considerably.

In wet AMD, because the oxygen supply to the macula is disrupted, the body responds by growing new, abnormal blood vessels. Older patients with this type of AMD can therefore experience a rapid change from healthy vision to severe visual impairment, leaving them little time to adjust. Inevitably the impact of such a diagnosis on quality of life can lead to depression. Periods of severe depression are not uncommon and are often made worse by the sleep deprivation that tends to accompany vision loss (Lewis & Southwell 2006). Information about the benefits of treatment may help to alleviate some of the feelings of depression.

Clearly, significant loss of vision has a substantial effect on quality of life and independent living, particularly for people who live alone (Watkinson & Scott 2010). Intra-vitreal anti-vascular endothelial growth factor therapy has advanced the treatment of wet AMD. Ranibizumab, 0.5mg, the drug of choice, is injected into the vitreous at the back of the eye to prevent degenerative blood vessels from growing and leaking (Watkinson & Scott 2010). Ranibizumab has been shown to stabilise sight in more than 90% of cases and improve sight in up to 40% (RNIB 2011).

Charles Bonnet Syndrome

Some older patients with AMD may experience Charles Bonnet Syndrome (CBS), in which visual hallucinations occur, resulting in anxiety and profound distress. Such experiences may also intensify any existing depression. A comprehensive explanation of this syndrome can reassure patients and help to relieve some of the visual distress. It should be emphasised that such experiences are a visual symptom and not a mental health problem, and that hallucinations usually seem to abate after 18 months for 60% of people (Ricard 2009). Importantly, providing such information may also help to avert further aggravation of the existing depression. Suggestions for controlling hallucinations include creating a brighter environment or a distraction, and looking directly at the images or making some form of eye movement (Ricard 2009).

Chronic open-angle glaucoma

Older people with COAG may become depressed when they are told that it is a chronic progressive disease for which there is no cure, and which is potentially blinding (Watkinson 2010). Once diagnosed, people with COAG will require lifelong monitoring to detect any progression of visual damage. Controlling the condition to prevent or minimise further damage is crucial to maintaining sight (NICE 2009b).

Adhering to prescribed treatment is important to maintain intra-ocular pressure within normal limits, preserve existing vision and prevent further visual loss (Watkinson 2010). However, poor adherence to therapy is common and well documented in patients with COAG (Gray et al. 2009, Olthoff et al. 2009). Depressive symptomatology and decreasing motivation levels only serve to intensify the poor adherence to treatment, with devastating outcomes for severe visual field and sight loss. Once sight has been lost, it cannot be recovered.

However, it is still important to stress that most people treated for COAG will not go blind (NICE 2009b). Barriers to adherence can be overcome by providing the older person and their family with the necessary information and support to develop good drop instillation techniques. This will help to reduce anxiety, promote self-confidence, alleviate some of the feelings of depression and provide a basis for longer-term independence. Good liaison with relatives can help optimise the older person's adherence to prescribed treatment.

Future perspectives

Clearly the key aim for the future is the development of routine screening for depression in older people with visual impairment. Already, NICE recommends screening high-risk groups for depression and providing treatment according to the 'stepped care' framework. However,

Margrain *et al.* (2012) contend that, although there is a high rate of depression in people with a visual disability, screening for depression and referral for treatment is not yet an integral part of visual rehabilitation service provision. One of the reasons advanced is that there may be no good evidence about the effectiveness of treatments in this patient group.

Margrain *et al.*'s (2012) study is the first to evaluate the effect of treatments for depression on people with a visual impairment and comorbid depression. This exploratory study, the Depression in Visual Impairment Trial (DEPVIT), will establish depression screening and referral for treatment in visual rehabilitation clinics in the UK. It is the first study to explore the efficacy of problem solving therapy (PST) and the effectiveness of NICE's 'stepped care' approach to the treatment of depression in people with a visual impairment.

Participants will be randomised to receive PST, a 'referral to the GP' requesting treatment according to the NICE's 'stepped care' recommendations, or placement on the waiting list arm of DEPVIT. The primary outcome measure is change in depressive symptoms, as measured by the Beck's Depression Inventory (BDI-II) at six months. Secondary outcomes include change in depressive symptoms at three months, change in visual function as measured with the near vision subscale of the VFQ-48 and seven-item NEI-VFQ at three and six months, change in generic health-related quality of life (EQ5D), the costs associated with PST, estimates of incremental cost-effectiveness, and recruitment rate estimation.

Conclusion

In summary, this chapter started by exploring the nature of depression and its classification as well as outlining its signs and symptoms, and the current key approaches to treatment. The role of the health and social care professional in the clinical management of depression in older people with visual impairment was then discussed, with specific reference to three major ocular diseases: cataract, AMD and COAG.

The primary challenge is to recognise the signs and symptoms of depression in older people with visual impairment and then to deliver the necessary help and emotional support, by means of psychosocial care, prior to further assessment and treatment. Accessing services for professional advice and continuing support will help the older person to regain better general and visual functioning and quality of life in the longer term.

Inevitably, the number of older people at risk of eye disease and its attendant complications will rise sharply over the next decade. Depression associated with sight loss is a burden to the older person and society in general and therefore warrants treatment on economic and moral grounds. The health and social care professional, as a health educator, can make a major contribution to the early detection of eye disease and assist in the prompt referral of older people for treatment and emotional support. This should help to avert some of the more distressing implications of sight loss, such as depression.

The key target for the future will be routine screening for depression in older people with the major ocular diseases discussed in this chapter. The theme of depression continues to be an issue for discussion in the following chapter, but this time with specific reference to visual impairment in older people with dementia.

References

Bambara, J., Owsley, C. & Wadley, V. (2009). Family caregiver social problem-solving abilities and adjustment to caring for a relative with vision loss. *Investigative Ophthalmology and Visual Science*. **50** (4), 1585–92.

Beck, A., Rush, A. & Shaw, B. (1979). *Cognitive Therapy of Depression*. New York. NY: The Guildford Press.

Blyth, C. (February 2006). Developments for MD patients – a clinician's update. *Journal of the Macular Disease Society. Digest*. 61–65.

Brody, B., Gamst, A. & Williams, R. (2001). Depression, visual acuity, comorbidity, and disability associated with age-related macular degeneration. *Ophthalmology*. **108** (10), 1893–901.

Department of Health (2011). *Talking Therapies: A Four-year Plan of Action. A Supporting Document to No Health Without Mental Health: A Cross-government Mental Health Outcomes Strategy for People of All Ages*. London: DH.

Evans, J., Fletcher, A. & Wormald, R. (2007). Depression and anxiety in visually impaired older people. *Ophthalmology*. **114** (2), 283–88.

Gray, T., Orton, L. & Henson, D. (2009). Interventions for improving adherence to ocular hypertensive therapy (Cochrane Review). *The Cochrane Library*. **2**. Chichester: Wiley-Blackwell.

Hayman, K., Kerse, N. & La Grow, S. (2007). Depression in older people: visual impairment and subjective ratings of health. *Optometry and Vision Science*. **84** (11), 1024–30.

Lewis, D. & Southwell, P. (February 2006). The psychological impact of MD – recurring themes. *Journal of the Macular Disease Society. Digest*. 35–37.

Mabuchi, F., Yoshimura, K. & Kashiwaqi, K. (2008). High prevalence of anxiety and depression in patients with primary open-angle glaucoma. *Journal of Glaucoma*. **17** (7), 552–57.

Margrain, T.H., Nollett, C. & Shearn, J. (2012). The Depression in Visual Impairment Trial (DEPVIT): trial design and protocol. *BMC Psychiatry*. **12**, 57.

Mental Health Foundation (2011). *Talking Therapies*. http://tinyurl.com/3cuzbq9 (Last accessed: 11 July 2012).

National Institute for Health and Clinical Excellence (2009a). *Depression: The Treatment and Management of Depression in Adults (Updated Edition)*. National Clinical Practice Guideline 90. London: NICE.

National Institute for Health and Clinical Excellence (2009b). *Glaucoma: Diagnosis and Management of Chronic Open-Angle Glaucoma and Ocular Hypertension*. Clinical Guideline 85. London: NICE.

National Institute for Health and Clinical Excellence (2011). *Quality Standard on Depression in Adults*. www.nice.org.uk/guidance/qualitystandards/depressioninadults/home.jsp (Last accessed: 11 July 2012).

Olthoff, C., Hoevenaars, J. & van den Borne, B. (2009). Prevalence and determinants of non-adherence to topical hypotensive treatment in Dutch glaucoma patients. *Graefe's Archive for Clinical and Experimental Ophthalmology*. **247** (2), 235–43.

Owsley, C., McGwin, G. Jr. & Scilley, K. (2007). Impact of cataract surgery on health-related quality of life in nursing home residents. *British Journal of Ophthalmology.* **91** (10), 1359–63.

Polack, S. (2008). Restoring sight: how cataract surgery improves the lives of older adults. *Community Eye Health.* **21** (66), 24–25.

Ricard, P. (2009). Vision loss and visual hallucinations: the Charles Bonnet Syndrome. *Community Eye Health.* **22** (69), 14.

Rovner, B., Casten, R. & Tasman, W. (2002). Effect of depression on visual function in age-related macular degeneration. *Archives of Ophthalmology.* **120** (8), 1041–44.

Roy, M., Roy, A. & Affouf, M. (2007). Depression is a risk factor for glycemic control and retinopathy in African-Americans with type 1 diabetes. *Psychosomatic Medicine.* **69** (6), 537–42.

Royal College of Psychiatrists (2011). 'Depression'. www.rcpsych.ac.uk/mentalhealthinfoforall/problems/depression/depression.aspx (Last accessed: 16 July 2012).

Royal National Institute of Blind People (2011). 'Anti-VEGF treatment for wet AMD'. www.rnib.org.uk/eye-health-eye-conditions-z-eye-conditions/anti-vegf-treatment (Last accessed: 8 May 2014).

Smith, D. (2009). 'Depression and Sight Loss'. Paper presented at the Wales and West Vision Conference Cardiff: Cardiff University.

Social Care Institute for Excellence (2006). *Assessing the Mental Health Needs of Older People. Adults' Services: SCIE Guide 03.* www.scie.org.uk/publications/guides/guide03/files/guide03.pdf (Last accessed: 16 July 2012).

Tod, A. (2011). A critique of positive thinking for patients with cancer. *Nursing Standard.* **25** (39), 43–47.

Unite for Sight (2011). Module 11: Eye Disease and Mental Health. www.uniteforsight.orh/community-eye-health-course/module11 (Last accessed: 24 April 2014).

Watkinson, S. (2010). Improving the care of chronic open-angle glaucoma. *Nursing Older People.* **22** (8), 18–23.

Watkinson, S. (2011). Managing depression in older people with visual impairment. *Nursing Older People.* **23** (8), 23–28.

Watkinson, S. & Scott, E. (2010). Care of patients undergoing intra-vitreal therapy. *Nursing Standard.* **24** (25), 42–47.

Wilkes, L., O'Baugh, J. & Luke, S. (2003). Positive attitude in cancer: patients' perspectives. *Oncology Nursing Forum.* **30** (3), 412–16.

World Health Organisation (2011). 'Depression'. www.who.int/topics/depression/en/ (Last accessed: 16 July 2012).

Chapter 9

Dementia and visually impaired older people

Susan Watkinson

This chapter covers

- Introduction
- Background to the condition
- What is dementia?
- Causes of dementia
- Risk factors
- Diagnosing dementia
- Alzheimer's disease: pathogenesis
- Visual changes in Alzheimer's disease
- Visual symptoms
- Specific visual difficulties in dementia
- Visual assessment
- Managing older people with dementia and visual impairment
- Future perspectives
- Conclusion

Introduction

This chapter discusses the care and management of older people with dementia and visual impairment. It begins with an overview of dementia, highlighting its nature, symptoms, the main types of dementia, and its diagnosis. Subsequently, the ocular effects associated with dementia and the importance of ocular examination will be explored, followed by a more in-depth discussion of some of the key visual and perceptual difficulties encountered by older people with dementia.

The management of older people with dementia and visual impairment will then be discussed in detail, with specific reference to the role and responsibilities of formal and informal carers. Finally, some future perspectives will be presented, in relation to the predicted social and economic implications of this condition in older people and the aims of ongoing research and training programmes.

Background to the condition

Dementia is one of the most severe and devastating disorders older people face (DH 2009). Its incidence and prevalence rise exponentially with age and it affects men and women in all social groups (DH 2009). There are currently 700,000 people with dementia in the United Kingdom (Alzheimer's Society 2012). By 2021, there will be over a million people with this disorder.

Currently, the national cost of this condition is about £17 billion per year (DH 2009). By 2038, the number of older people with dementia is expected to double to 1.4 million and the national cost to rise to over £50 billion per year (DH 2009).

Older Black, Asian and minority ethnic people

An increase in the number of older Black, Asian and minority ethnic (BAME) people in the UK is likely to lead to an increased need for dementia services. The latest evidence suggests that there are nearly 25,000 people with dementia from BAME communities and this number is set to increase seven-fold to over 170,000 by 2051 (All-Party Parliamentary Group on Dementia 2013).

Currently, BAME people are under-represented in dementia services and this is largely due to lower levels of awareness of dementia, the existence of stigma within the BAME communities, and a lack of appropriate support (Moriarty et al. 2011). There needs to be an improved uptake of services, and it may be possible to achieve this by developing information resources and appointing workers with responsibility for outreach programmes.

Clearly, more training is required for staff working in dementia services to facilitate more effective delivery of culturally acceptable care and support to BAME people with dementia (Moriarty et al. 2011). Carers of BAME older people with dementia may be reluctant to ask for help, although support (such as carers' groups and respite services) may be appreciated. It is also important to remember that different communities may have differing views about whether they wish these services to be culturally specific or mixed.

The National Dementia Strategy

Since the advent of the National Dementia Strategy (DH 2009), the government has been committed to improving the care and experience of older people with dementia and their carers. The strategy set out a vision for transforming dementia services to achieve better awareness, early diagnosis and high-quality treatment at every stage and in every setting, with greater focus on local delivery of quality outcomes and local accountability for achieving them. Providing specialist care to improve eye health screening and low vision services continues to be a priority for the government, according to the UK Vision Strategy (RNIB 2013).

An increasing number of older people with dementia may develop visual impairment, since sight loss is largely an age-related phenomenon. Although, this is a current concern (Watkinson 2009), no reference has been made to the need for eye care provision in the National Dementia Strategy for England (DH 2009). The diagnosis of dementia and sight loss is nevertheless important in order to ensure high-quality treatment and care of the individual, as deprivation profoundly advances the sense of disorientation (Jones & Trigg 2007). Other problems associated with dementia – such as communication issues, difficulty with daily living activities, and depression – will also be compounded by failing vision (Watkinson 2009).

The co-existence of diagnosed dementia and age-related visual impairment will become increasingly important in the future, especially in view of demographic change. Currently, there is a low level of diagnosis and treatment of dementia in the UK, with a 24-fold variation between highest and lowest activity by primary care trust (DH 2009). In fact, only 43% of people with dementia in the UK receive a diagnosis (Alzheimer's Society 2012). Indeed, international comparisons suggest that the UK is in the bottom third of European performance in terms of diagnosis and treatment, with less than half the activity of France, Sweden, Ireland and Spain (DH 2009). Overall, the number of older people with dementia is steadily increasing and careful planning is critical to ensure that services are available to provide the right care and support for the future.

What is dementia?

The term 'dementia' is used to describe the symptoms that occur when the brain is affected by specific diseases and conditions (Alzheimer's Society 2012). Dementia is progressive, which means that symptoms gradually get worse over time. The rate at which dementia progresses depends on the individual and the type of dementia diagnosed. Each person's experience of dementia is unique (Alzheimer's Society 2012) and the symptoms are listed in Table 9.1 (page 154).

Table 9.1: Symptoms of dementia

Loss of memory	Affects short-term memory in particular. Examples are:
	● Forgetting what happened earlier in the day
	● Inability to recall conversations
	● Repeating oneself
	● Forgetting the way home from the shops.
	Long-term memory is usually quite good.
Mood changes	The person may be withdrawn, sad, frightened or angry about what is happening to them.
Communication problems	Difficulty finding the right words for things – for example, describing the function of an item instead of naming it.
	A decline in the ability to read and write.

(Adapted from Alzheimer's Society 2012)

Causes of dementia

There are several diseases and conditions that can result in dementia. The most common are Alzheimer's disease and vascular dementia. The others are included in Table 9.2 opposite.

Risk factors

Age is the most significant risk factor for dementia. One in 50 people aged between 65 and 70 years has some form of dementia. One in five people aged over 80 years has dementia (Alzheimer's Society, 2012).

This increased risk may be due to hypertension, the increased incidence of some diseases, such as heart disease and stroke, changes to nerve cells, DNA and cell structure, and the weakening of natural repair systems (Alzheimer's Society 2012). Overall, the risk of developing dementia depends on a combination of genetic and environmental factors. Table 9.3 (page 155) details the specific risk factors. With reference to the genetic factor, those thought to have a genetic cause of dementia and their unaffected relatives should be offered referral for genetic counselling (NICE 2011).

Vascular dementia is thought to be more common among Asian and Black Caribbean people because they are more prone to risk factors for vascular dementia such as cardiovascular disease, hypertension and diabetes (Moriarty *et al.* 2011).

Table 9.2: Causes of dementia

Alzheimer's disease	Most common cause Chemistry and structure of brain change, leading to death of brain cells Short-term memory loss – usually the first noticeable sign.
Vascular dementia	Brain cells die due to lack of oxygen caused by vascular disease Symptoms may occur suddenly following a stroke, or over time following a series of small strokes.
Dementia with Lewy bodies	Tiny abnormal structures develop inside nerve cells, leading to degeneration of brain tissue. Symptoms include disorientation, hallucinations and difficulties with planning, reasoning and problem-solving Memory may be affected to a lesser degree Shares some characteristics with Parkinson's disease.
Frontal-temporal dementia	Damage usually focused in the front part of the brain Personality and behavioural changes are the most obvious signs.

(Adapted from Alzheimer's Society 2012)

Table 9.3: Specific risk factors associated with dementia

Risk factor	Details
Gender	• Women are slightly more likely to develop Alzheimer's disease (AD) than men. • Men more commonly develop vascular dementia (VD).
Genetics	• Hereditary diseases that may cause dementia include Huntington's disease, Familial AD (very rare), Niemann-Pick Type C disease. • Certain genes, such as apolipoprotein E (ApoE), are involved in the development of AD and VD.

cont.

Medical history	• Specific medical conditions can increase the risk of dementia. These include: multiple sclerosis, Huntington's disease, Down's syndrome and human immunodeficiency virus (HIV).
	• Mid-life hypertension, high blood cholesterol levels, stroke, heart attack and irregular heart rhythms increase the risk of VD.
	• Mid-life obesity can increase the risk of dementia.
	• Severe or repeated head injuries can increase the risk of dementia.
Diet	• Too much saturated fat increases the risk of heart attacks, stroke and vascular disease, which can lead to VD.
Smoking	• Smoking has extremely harmful effects on the heart, lungs and vascular system, including blood vessels in the brain. It increases the risk of VD.
Alcohol	• Drinking excessive amounts of alcohol over a long period of time increases the risk of developing Korsakoff's syndrome.
Physical exercise	• A good level of physical health helps to protect against dementia.
	• Regular physical exercise helps to reduce the risk of developing VD.

(Adapted from the Alzheimer's Society website, 2012)

Diagnosing dementia

Diagnosing dementia is often very difficult, especially in the early stages. Initially, the older person should consult the GP who may then refer them to a specialist consultant for confirmation of diagnosis.

Assessments may include conversations with the older person and close family members, a physical examination, memory tests and/or brain scans (Alzheimer's Society 2012). The Mini Mental State Examination (MMSE) is the most commonly used test for complaints related to memory problems or when a diagnosis of dementia is being considered.

Memory loss can be the outcome of ageing, so forgetfulness does not necessarily signal dementia in the older person (Alzheimer's Society 2012). Memory loss can also be a symptom of stress or depression. In rarer cases, dementia-like symptoms can be caused by vitamin deficiencies or a brain tumour.

Disturbances of the visual system can pre-date other manifestations of dementia. However, diagnosis may be overlooked due to characteristic vague symptomatology and normal eyesight examination findings at presentation (Shayler 2011). Older patients with AD usually seek an ophthalmic consultation because of disturbances of pattern processing and recognition.

Alzheimer's disease: pathogenesis

As AD is the most common cause of dementia among older people, it is useful to give a brief overview of its pathogenesis as a basis for understanding the older person's symptoms. In AD, there is a deposit of abnormal protein outside nerve cells in the form of amyloid.

These are called diffuse plaques. The amyloid also forms the core of more organised plaques called senile or neurotic plaques. There is an accumulation of abnormal filaments called neurofibrillary tangles. There can also be atrophy of the affected areas of the brain and enlargement of the ventricles, as well as loss of the neurotransmitters serotonin, acetylcholine, norepinephrine and somatostatin (Solomons 2005).

Visual changes in Alzheimer's disease

Older people with dementia can experience a number of visual perceptual difficulties due to normal ageing, eye conditions, and sometimes from additional damage to the visual system caused by specific types of dementia (Alzheimer's Society 2012). In fact, more than 60% of people with AD have a decline in one or more visual functions (Shayler 2011).

AD causes vision impairment through deterioration of neurological function within the brain, and not by affecting the eye. As previously indicated, the 'plaque and tangle' damage, which characterises AD, initially accumulates in areas of the brain linked to memory for processing new factual information. It is also situated close to a part of the visual pathway, which can also become affected by the spread of plaque and tangles.

Subsequently, other parts of the visual pathway can become involved. Difficulties in both primary and complex visual functioning have been documented for AD (Alzheimer's Society 2012).

Visual symptoms

Difficulty with near reading is the most common symptom and may present as skipping of words or lines on a page, 'dancing print' (a form of acquired visual dyslexia) and/or blurred vision. The latter can progress to alexia in advanced disease (Shayler 2011). See Table 9.4 (page 158) for some of the other typical visual symptoms experienced in AD.

Table 9.4: Typical visual symptoms experienced in AD

- Vision deteriorates under stress
- Blurred vision at distance, intermediate (such as computer screens), and/or near, which is not fully relieved with spectacles
- Problems with judging depth
- Eye strain with no apparent cause
- Slow reading
- Loss of concentration when reading
- 'Can't be bothered' with reading small print
- Driving a car causes strain or tired eyes
- Light sensitivity
- Restricted depth of focus when reading
- Eyes 'just don't seem quite right'
- Balance and/or postural problems
- Clumsiness, falls, walking into objects and/or knocking over ornaments.

(Adapted from Shayler 2011)

The specific visual difficulties encountered in AD are listed in Table 9.5 below.

Table 9.5: Specific visual difficulties in AD

- Fewer and less accurate small eye movements
- Colour perception (loss of blue, purple and green part of the spectrum)
- Figure–background contrast discrimination
- Depth and motion perception
- Visual acuity (not initially)
- Object and facial recognition.

(Adapted from Alzheimer's Society 2012)

Visual assessment

The visual assessment of people with dementia can be complicated because it is often difficult to distinguish the effects of dementia on basic visual function from its effects on higher cognitive function. Moreover, poor cognition can lead to poor performance in visual tests and, conversely, poor vision can produce poor performance in cognitive tests (Thomas Pocklington Trust 2010). However, patients with dementia who are failing to have regular eye examinations are a cause for concern, as they consequently risk sight loss from typical age-related sight problems such as cataract, glaucoma and age-related macular degeneration.

Assessment and treatment of these conditions can improve balance, posture, walking ability, visual aspects of motion awareness, contrast, visual acuity and colour vision (Shayler 2011). This, in turn, leads to improved ability to read and watch TV, for example, and, more importantly, enhances quality of life.

Managing older people with dementia and visual impairment

It has been estimated that at least 2.5% of people aged over 75 have both dementia and serious visual impairment. Furthermore, the combined effects of these conditions can severely restrict independence. This results in an increased reliance on family carers and a higher risk of institutionalisation (Lawrence et al. 2008). Alarmingly, however, evidence suggests that some healthcare professionals attach minimal significance to sight loss, describing their work as holistic – in terms of meeting multiple needs and expressing less concern about working with older people with both dementia and sight loss. In addition, few healthcare professionals feel that sight loss has a significant effect on the way they work with clients (Lawrence et al. 2008).

It is therefore critically important for both formal and family carers to understand that the experience of joint sight loss and dementia creates a profound sense of disorientation in older people. Many have difficulty recalling the time and their surroundings, and are unable to locate themselves using visual cues. This often results in distress and occasionally leads to agitated and aggressive behaviour (Lawrence et al. 2008). Significantly, there is evidence that such disorientation can also result in falls (Allan et al. 2009).

The role of formal carers is to meet the needs of older people and their family carers in order to reduce the impact of serious sight loss and dementia on quality of life. The following discussion therefore focuses on some of the key care interventions that provide practical support to achieve a safer environment and improved quality of life for the older person with this dual loss. Formal and informal carers in primary and secondary healthcare and social settings should recognise that sight loss creates needs that require extra time and attention.

If older people are to be supported in a way that promotes (rather than undermines) their autonomy, it is essential for all carers to meet these needs.

Eye care and visual health

Firstly, the older person should be encouraged to wear spectacles, if needed, to improve their overall visual acuity. It is also essential to ensure that the older person is wearing the glasses required for a specific task (RNIB 2014). For example, reading glasses must be worn for close tasks, and distance glasses for all other activities. It is helpful to label glasses so that everyone can distinguish between those for reading and distance. If glasses are worn by an older person, it is equally important for the carer to check that they are clean – to facilitate clearer vision.

Similarly, it is important to check that the older person's lens prescription is still effective in correcting any existing refractive errors. This will necessitate the arranging of regular eye checks. If the older person is in a more advanced stage of dementia, special non-verbal tests (as used for people with learning difficulties) may be required.

In general, it is important to remember that glasses cannot correct difficulties resulting from other types of damage to the visual system, such as cataracts, age-related macular degeneration or retinal detachment. For example, if cataracts are found to be a contributory cause of poor sight, the older person must be referred to the GP for treatment. It is helpful for a family member to communicate, with the older person's consent, any sight problems the older person may have. The approach to caring and the adjustments required to meet the older person's sight needs, should be clearly documented in the daily care plan (RNIB 2014).

Managing visual hallucinations

It is acknowledged that older people with dementia are less able to express their needs and are more likely to have uncorrected visual deficits (Lawrence et al. 2008). Evidence has also shown that poor vision in people with dementia not only leads to an accelerated loss of independence but also an increased risk of psychotic symptoms such as visual hallucinations. The latter are common and disruptive (Lawrence et al. 2008).

Carers, particularly family members, often need guidance on how to manage the older person's visual hallucinations. They should try to reduce the individual's feelings of distress by offering support and reassurance and being non-confrontational. Exploring hallucinations and explaining what is happening can sometimes help older people make sense of their experience. The use of distraction techniques to focus the older person's attention elsewhere can also be useful. Encourage eye movements, and create the opposite situation. For example, if hallucinations usually occur in bright light, try dimming the lights. Conversely, it may be beneficial to reduce shadows and improve lighting (RNIB 2014).

Promoting a safe environment

Older people with dementia can be helped by aiding specific visual functions. For example, improving lighting levels can help to achieve this (Jones & van der Eerden 2008). It is estimated that more than half of British homes do not have enough lighting even for ordinary purposes. Improved lighting has also been found to be instrumental in preventing falls and reducing visual hallucinations. Overall, it is essential to provide good even lighting and try to eliminate shadows. Making environmental adaptations may be necessary, such as removing 'busy' patterns on walls, furniture or floors, which tend to create visual clutter, and removing shiny surfaces which cause glare (RNIB 2014). In addition, changes in floor surfaces or patterns can exacerbate visuoperceptual difficulties.

Minimising visual and physical obstacles is therefore beneficial. Slip and trip hazards can also be reduced by helping older people to put things away and find them easily again, using clear storage containers and/or labelling (RNIB 2014).

The deliberate use of colour cues and contrasts to make different areas or items clear can help significantly. For example, a white plate on a white tablecloth can be difficult to find. Similarly, white doors in white walls make it hard to locate rooms or cupboards. Dunne et al. (2004) showed that for people with advanced AD changing to highly visible red cups and plates led to a 25% increase in food intake and an 84% increase in liquid consumption.

Brightly coloured toilet doors have also been used successfully in a variety of care settings to help older people with dementia find the toilet independently and more readily. Additionally, high colour contrast toilet seats can make it easier to locate them. If a person needs handrails, it is advisable to choose extra-long ones so that they are as conspicuous as possible (Alzheimer's Society 2012). Making routes between different rooms or places clear by using easily visible signs, which contrast with their surroundings, is also important. Assistive technologies, ranging from automatic lights to audio labels, can also be very helpful.

Such practical support is vital in order to maintain a safe environment and reduce the risk of falls and consequent injuries. Falls are a major cause of morbidity and mortality in dementia (Allan et al. 2009). Older people with dementia recover less well after a fall than those without dementia. Preventing falls is therefore an urgent priority for carers both in the community and in hospital settings. Allan et al. (2009) found that for older people with dementia living in the community the incidence of falls was ten times higher than for those without dementia. Significantly, the annual incidence of falls was higher in those with Dementia with Lewy Bodies (DLB) and Parkinson's disease with dementia (PDD) than in all other groups studied. Moreover, the incidence of falls was higher in those with PDD than DLB (Allan et al. 2009).

Reducing disorientation and increasing independence

Formal and informal carers need to provide clear, regular communication to promote the older person's sense of orientation and confidence in their environment. Techniques such as reality orientation and validation therapy may help to raise older people's awareness of external reality (Lawrence *et al.* 2008).

It is therefore important to talk to older people with dementia and sight loss about what is happening to and around them. The carer should always be able to explain where they are going and describe the route while walking along. This should help to reduce their sense of disorientation and increase their independence. Similarly, at mealtimes, describing the food and drink being offered, where it is positioned on the table, and who or what is beside or nearby, can be helpful.

Overall, older people need to know where their personal belongings are, and feel reassured that they are where they left them. Leaving items as the older person left them can support independence (RNIB 2014). It is also important to tell an older person with sight loss whenever you are entering or leaving the room. Equally, explanation is beneficial when administering medication, or supporting an older person to take their own medication. Explaining what is happening, and what the medicine is for, can enhance the older person's compliance with prescribed therapy.

Reducing loneliness and isolation

Older people with dementia and sight loss often experience loneliness and isolation (Lawrence *et al.* 2008). Clearly, the combination of sight and memory loss restricts their participation in hobbies and social groups. The carer should adopt some practical approaches to identify stimulating activities that are accessible to older people in this situation. The aim is to provide engaging and interesting activities. Such activities might include keeping up to date with the news via talking newspapers, listening to audio books, and film and TV audio description. Tactile or large-print games or making music choices (via audio labels) are also engaging activities for older people to pursue. Evidence suggests that older people with sight and memory loss enjoy spending time with others who have similar conditions (Lawrence *et al.* 2008). They may enjoy group activities such as singing and dancing, cookery and food tasting.

Overall, the use of scent, sound, touch and movement can be therapeutic. If the older person is visiting a place of interest, audio descriptions can be found or created to enhance their experience and enjoyment of it. For any activity, giving clear information about what is going on and providing encouragement and support will facilitate the older person's enjoyment and involvement.

Conversely, many older people are only able to cope with one-to-one interaction and are very dependent on their carers for stimulation (Lawrence *et al.* 2008). Clearly, this group of older people would benefit from more one-to-one contact with paid carers and volunteers, especially if more time could be devoted to maintaining their pastimes. However, it is often the case in care homes, for example, that limited resources restrict opportunities for one-to-one contact. Nonetheless, it remains critically important that the value of such contact for this client group is appreciated.

Supporting family carers

Family carers face a great many daily challenges and exceptional demands. In view of this, it is very helpful to provide them with information about the resources that are available to help with the older person's dementia and sight loss. For example, night carers may be necessary, and more sessions at day centres may be required as a means of providing extra respite. Some family carers may also become depressed, due to the psychological demands of intensive caring.

Indeed, NICE (2011) recommends that carers of people with dementia who experience psychological distress and negative psychological impact should be offered psychological therapy, including cognitive behavioural therapy, conducted by a specialist. Family carers should also contact their primary care physician to get information about the counselling services that are available. It is essential to support family members in this difficult and emotionally traumatic situation, and they should also be informed about the useful fact sheets produced by the Alzheimer's Society and the RNIB. Table 9.5 lists additional resources that could be explored.

Table 9.5: Additional resources for family carers

Information about dementia

- Alzheimer's Society: www.alzheimers.org.uk
- Alzheimer's Society book of activities (Knocker 2003)
- Hallucinations in people with dementia: www.alzheimers.org.uk/factsheet/520
- Visuoperceptual difficulties in dementia: www.alzheimers.org.uk/factsheet/527

Information and advice about sight loss

- RNIB: www.rnib.org.uk for practical support, information, and local resource centres
- Local sight loss charities: www.visionary.org.uk
- Disability equipment centres: www.assist-org.uk

cont.

- Thomas Pocklington Trust: www.pocklington-trust.org.uk for housing and lighting; good practice guides
- Macular Disease Society: www.maculardisease.org for information about the most common cause of sight loss in older people in the UK.

Future perspectives

Demographics and financial costs

Over the next three decades, the challenges of an ageing UK society will demand that services be prepared to assess and treat increasing numbers of older people with both dementia and sight loss. Older people with dementia are clearly less able to cope with the added burden of visual impairment. Their reduced sight will impact greatly on their cognitive performance, mobility and daily living activities. Inevitably, this will have implications for the government in meeting the costs of care, support and treatment in the longer term for this psychologically complex, demanding and vulnerable group of people and their family carers.

Economic climate and nurse training

Bearing in mind the current climate of economic austerity, the UK government will probably struggle to meet key priorities for the healthcare of older people with dementia and sight loss over the next decade. Already, financial restraints have resulted in reduced numbers of registered nurses, a recent decline in nurse training, and, significantly, increasing angst expressed by the nursing profession about falling standards of care for older people. Greater numbers of healthcare assistants and support workers are being employed as a way of repairing the nursing deficit. This practice is currently embedding within NHS culture and is likely to remain the cheaper option for providing basic care for the foreseeable future.

Importance of regular eye examinations

Regular eye examinations are important for people with dementia, as these individuals are potentially more at risk of visual impairment than people without dementia. Improving the uptake of sight tests would be a positive step towards improving their eye health. More research needs to be done on this subject, as limited data currently exists on the level of uptake and frequency of sight tests among people with dementia.

Raising awareness

For the future, it is essential to raise awareness among people with dementia and their carers of the fact that dementia is strongly linked to a potential decline in vision and eye health. Carers should be helped to access information and advice from websites in order to understand the vision problems associated with dementia, and the concurrence of dementia and certain eye conditions. Similarly, it would be advantageous to provide online education and training resources for all carers of older people with dementia and sight loss.

Conclusion

In summary, this chapter has addressed the management of older people with dementia and sight loss. Initially, the background to dementia in the UK was presented. An overview of dementia was then provided, with reference to the underlying pathophysiological changes and the clinical symptoms emerging as a result. The causes and main types of dementia were identified and the risk factors and current methods of diagnosis were outlined. Subsequently, the visual changes taking place in Alzheimer's disease and the resulting visual symptoms were described, and the specific visual difficulties experienced by people with Alzheimer's disease were outlined. Reference was then made to some of the difficulties involved in visually assessing older people with dementia.

This chapter presented an in-depth discussion of the management of older people with dementia and visual impairment particularly regarding the role of formal and informal carers in primary and secondary healthcare, and social settings. In summary, identifying and addressing the key aspects of care and practical support required to meet the needs of this group of older people is a vital means of reducing the impact of dementia and serious sight loss on quality of life.

Because of the complexity of caring for this group of older people, an integrated approach to the management and delivery of care is vital. Consequently, visual rehabilitation and mental health teams and voluntary sector agencies can work with other carers to provide maximum benefit for older people. It is equally important to ensure that all contributors to care have access to dementia-care training and skill development order to facilitate more effective management of the unique challenges posed by the co-existence of dementia and visual impairment in this vulnerable group of people.

The next and final chapter in the book will present a summary of current and future perspectives on the clinical management and care of older people with visual impairment.

References

Allan, L.M., Ballard, C.G., Rowan, E.N. & Kenny, R.A. (2009). Incidence and Prediction of Falls in Dementia: A Prospective Study in Older People. *PLoS ONE*. **4** (5), e5521. www.plosone.org/article/info%3Adoi%2F10.1371%2Fjournal.pone.0005521#pone-000521.g002 (Last accessed: 28 April 2014).

All-Party Parliamentary Group on Dementia (July 2013). *Dementia does not discriminate. The experiences of black, Asian, and minority ethnic communities.* APPG. www.alzheimers.org.uk/site/scripts/download_info.php?downloadID=1186 (Last accessed: 19 January 2014).

Alzheimer's Society (2012): 'What is dementia?' www.alzheimers.org.uk/site/scripts/documents_info.php?documentID=106 (Last accessed: 3 August 2012).

Department of Health (2009). *Living Well with Dementia: A National Dementia Strategy.* London: DH.

Dunne, T.E., Neargarder, S.A., Cippolloni, P. & Cronin-Golomb, A. (2004). Visual contrast enhances food and liquid intake in advanced Alzheimer's disease. *Clinical Nutrition.* **23**, 533–38.

Jones, G.M.M. & van der Eerden, W.J. (2008). Designing care environments for persons with Alzheimer's dementia: visuoperceptual considerations. *Reviews in Clinical Gerontology.* **18**, 13–37.

Jones, R. & Trigg, R. (2007). *Dementia and Serious Sight Loss.* Occasional Paper, No. 11. London: Thomas Pocklington Trust.

Knocker, S. (2003). Alzheimer's Society book of activities. Food, fun and parties. www.alzheimers.org.uk/site/scripts/press_article.php?pressReleaseID=21 (Last accessed: 28 April 2014).

Lawrence, V., Murray, J., Ffytche, D. & Banerjee, S. (2008). *The experiences and needs of people with dementia and serious visual impairment: a qualitative study.* Occasional Paper 16 (November). London: Thomas Pocklington Trust.

Moriarty, L., Sharif, N. & Robinson, J. (2011). *Black and minority ethnic people with dementia and their access to support and services.* Research Briefing 35. www.scie.org.uk/publications/briefings/files/briefing35.pdf (Last accessed: 19 January 2014).

National Institute for Health and Clinical Excellence (2011). *Dementia: Supporting people with dementia and their carers in health and social care. Clinical Guideline No 42.* London: NICE.

Royal National Institute of Blind People (2013). UK Vision Strategy 2013–2018 Vision 2020 UK. www.vision2020uk.org.uk/ukvisionstrategy/core/core_picker/download.asp?id=539&filetitle=UK+Vision (Last accessed: 28 April 2014).

Royal National Institute of Blind People (2014). 'Dementia and sight loss'. www.rnib.org.uk/eye-health-sight-loss-other-medical-conditions/dementia-and-sight-loss (Last accessed: 28 April 2014).

Shayler, G. (2011). Vision dysfunction in Alzheimer's Disease. Ageing Vision Part 3, Course Code: C-15561 0. Ot CET: 41–49. www.optometry.co.uk/uploads/articles/cet_1-110211.pdf (Last accessed: 20 September 2012).

Solomons, H. (October 2005). Vision and dementia. *Optometry.* 25–28.

Thomas Pocklington Trust (2010). *Improving vision and eye healthcare to people with dementia.* Research Discussion Paper, Number 8, 1–7. London: Thomas Pocklington Trust.

Watkinson, S. (2009). Visual Impairment in Older People. *Nursing Older People.* **21** (8), 30–36.

Chapter 10

Conclusion

Susan Watkinson

This chapter covers

- Introduction
- Demographic change and health policy
- Epidemiology of sight loss
- Economic impact of sight loss
- Psychosocial impact of sight loss
- Age-related ocular disease
- The future role of health and social care professionals
- Conclusion

Introduction

This book has considered the management of older people with visual impairment due to the major age-related ocular diseases in the UK. It has also examined some of the significant issues influencing this area of practice: namely, demographic change, health policy, the epidemiology of sight loss, the impact of sight loss on the UK economy, and the psychosocial impact of visual impairment and the way it can reduce quality of life for older people.

In relation to the main ocular diseases, the health and social care professional's role was discussed in detail, particularly what is expected from healthcare professionals in terms of contributing to the care of older people in the UK for the future. Importantly, each chapter presented the current approaches to treatment of the specific ocular disease under review. Furthermore, where relevant, future perspectives on treatment (based on advancing technology and a newly emerging research evidence base) were outlined.

Demographic change and health policy

Demographic change is probably the most significant issue facing the UK for the remainder of the twenty-first century. By 2031, it is predicted that 27.2 million people will be over the age of 50. Furthermore, in the next 30 years, people aged 85 and over will constitute 3.8% of the UK population (Office for National Statistics 2009). Such projections will inevitably mean an increase in the incidence of visual impairment, as sight loss is largely an age-related phenomenon.

More significantly, recent evidence suggests that the estimated numbers of older people with dementia in Black, Asian and minority ethnic (BAME) groups in England and Wales will be far higher than previously thought. A seven-fold increase in their numbers is expected, compared with a two-fold increase in the rest of the population. It has been suggested that this significant increase is due to that fact that immigrants who came to the UK in the 1950s and 1970s are now reaching their seventh and eighth decades.

As previously highlighted in Chapter 9, there are lower levels of awareness about dementia and a stigma about dementia within BAME communities. The All-Parliamentary Group on Dementia is therefore calling for Public Health England to fund a pilot awareness campaign to inform minority ethnic communities about the condition and at the same time challenge the existing stigma (Alzheimer's Society 2013).

Generally, the demand for eye services will increase and eye care will need to be regarded as an integral part of healthcare for all older people. In the current UK Vision Strategy 2013–2018 (RNIB 2013a), three major strategy outcomes are identified for eye health and sight loss services over the next five years, as follows:

Outcome 1: Everyone in the UK looks after their eyes and their sight.

Outcome 2: Everyone with an eye condition receives timely treatment and, if permanent sight loss occurs, early and appropriate services and support are available to all.

Outcome 3: We have a society in which people with sight loss can fully participate.

Providing specialist care to improve eye health screening and low vision services must remain a priority. However, there is still cause for concern about the increasing number of older people with dementia who may develop visual impairment, and the National Dementia Strategy for England (DH 2009) makes no reference to their need for eye care provision.

Epidemiology of sight loss

Currently, almost two million people in the UK are living with sight loss, which amounts to approximately one person in 30 (RNIB 2013b). Because of our ageing population, the number of people with sight loss is set to increase dramatically in the future (RNIB 2013a). Furthermore, there is a growing incidence of key underlying causes of sight loss, such as diabetes and obesity (RNIB 2013b). It is therefore predicted that in the UK, by 2020, the number of people with sight loss will have risen to 2,250,000. By 2050, this number will have doubled to nearly four million (RNIB 2013a). Significantly, 50% of sight loss can be avoided through preventative action, and this strengthens the case for more intensive public health education.

Economic impact of sight loss

Inevitably, expenditure on eye care and treatment will rise with the predicted increase in sight loss (RNIB 2013a). Costs related to the four main age-related ocular diseases addressed in this book are substantial. For example, in 2010 £129 million was spent on Lucentis, the current treatment of choice for wet age-related macular degeneration (AMD), making it the fourth most costly drug prescribed across all areas of the NHS in England (NHSIC 2011a). Also, in 2010 a total of £129 million was spent on glaucoma prescriptions. This figure relates only to the community, and does not include hospital-dispensed prescriptions. In total, glaucoma prescriptions represent around two-thirds of all expenditure on eye health prescriptions dispensed in the community (NHSIC 2011c).

With reference to cataract services, removal of cataract is the most common surgical intervention performed in the NHS in England. In the UK, approximately 400,000 NHS cataract operations were undertaken in 2010 and 2011. Each cataract operation costs the NHS £932. However, by way of comparison, this is cheaper than repairing a fractured hip, which costs £9000, and in older people is frequently due to a fall that is related to visual impairment (NHSIC 2011b).

Retinal screening is pivotal to detecting the early pathophysiological changes taking place in the retinal capillaries in diabetic retinopathy. However, only 79% of patients who were offered diabetic retinopathy screening took part in the NHS retinal screening programme (National Screening Committee 2012).

Psychosocial impact of sight loss

As highlighted in Chapter 1, visual impairment can have a substantial detrimental effect on the psychosocial status of individuals and their quality of life, often leading to isolation and depression (RNIB 2009). Isolation is a particularly high risk for blind and partially sighted older people. For example, the more severe older people's sight loss is, the higher the probability that they will never leave their homes (RNIB 2013b). Furthermore, almost 50% of people who report poor vision or blindness confirm that they always deliberately limit the amount of walking they do outside their house. This compares to 12% of people with good or better vision who confirm the same behaviour (RNIB 2013b). Many blind and partially sighted people also face social exclusion, and 44% report that they feel moderately or completely cut off from people and things around them (RNIB 2013b).

The link between sight loss and reduced psychosocial well-being, particularly for older people, is clear; around 35% of older people with sight loss also have some form of depression (RNIB 2013b). The primary challenge for all health and social care professionals is to recognise the signs and symptoms of depression in older people with visual impairment and to deliver the necessary psychosocial help and emotional support before arranging further assessment and treatment. Depression associated with sight loss is a burden both to the older person and society in general, and treatment is therefore justified on both economic and moral grounds.

Age-related ocular disease

Cataract, age-related macular degeneration (AMD), chronic open-angle glaucoma (COAG) and diabetic retinopathy remain the most significant ocular conditions affecting older people in the UK.

Visual impairment due to cataract can have a major negative impact on the quality of older people's lives and can result in difficulties with daily living activities (Polack 2008). It is therefore important to dispel the misconception that sight is less important in older age and that the restrictive impact of vision loss should be accepted as part of the ageing process (Polack 2008).

AMD is the leading cause of irreversible blindness in people over 50 years of age in the Western world. In the UK, it accounts for more than half of all registered blindness and there is still no cure for this condition (Kanski & Bowling 2011).

COAG is a chronic condition that affects older people and requires lifetime monitoring and management. It affects approximately 480,000 people in the UK and there are over a million glaucoma-related hospital outpatient visits annually (NICE 2009). After AMD, it is one of the principal reasons for having to register as blind (NICE 2009).

Diabetes mellitus is one of the biggest health challenges facing the UK today. By 2025, it is estimated that five million people will have diabetes. Most of these cases will be type 2 diabetes, because of an ageing population and rapidly rising numbers of overweight and obese people (Diabetes UK 2012). Similarly, the numbers of people with eye disease such as diabetic retinopathy will also increase. Diabetic retinopathy is currently a major cause of blindness in people with diabetes and remains one of the leading causes of blindness in the Western world (Riordan-Eva & Whitcher 2008).

Good metabolic control, as discussed in Chapter 5, can help to delay the onset and progression of diabetic retinopathy. Furthermore, early detection and treatment of vision-threatening retinopathy can help to prevent or delay blindness. Importantly, however, this involves regular eye examinations and timely intervention (WHO 2013). Thus, retinal screening is pivotal to an effective prevention strategy.

External eye disease

In addition to the main intra-ocular diseases addressed in this text, Chapter 6 discussed several external ocular conditions that commonly occur in older people. Such external eye disease was highlighted as being equally distressing and uncomfortable in terms of disturbed vision and reduced quality of life. Accurate diagnosis of the presenting condition is therefore required, and appropriate care and treatment must be given in order to promote good vision and comfortable eyes.

The future role of health and social care professionals

The role will be directed and supported towards creating the right culture within the NHS, which is seen to be pivotal to achieving high-quality care. This is in the wake of a three-year vision and strategy for nursing, midwifery and care staff, which is aiming to build a culture of compassion in all areas of practice (DH 2012).

The expected values and behaviours of healthcare workers are embodied in the 6 Cs, which are perceived to be the cornerstone of patient-centred care; these are care, compassion, competence, courage and commitment (DH 2012). Such values and behaviour will be particularly important in handling the care and management of older people in the future. With specific reference to older people, similar guidelines have previously been provided for healthcare professionals. They emphasise safe and effective quality care, and promoting the older person's dignity by nurturing self-respect and self-worth (NMC 2009).

In the current climate, such guidelines serve as a timely reminder that good healthcare and support systems are not universal and that examples of very poor care have recently been witnessed within the NHS (DH 2013). Of the 290 recommendations made by the Francis Report, one of the most significant was the need for improved support for compassionate, caring, committed nursing and stronger leadership (DH 2013). Clearly, looking after older people will present many challenges for developing the caring role in practice. This is especially true of older people with visual impairment, and the need to meet the growing demands placed on both primary and community-based eye health services (Watkinson 2009). In the future, ophthalmic nurses and other relevant health and social care professionals will need to continue to deliver high-quality care for older people with visual impairment (Watkinson 2009).

Competence

Technological advances, specialist ophthalmic nurses, and the competent delivery of technical skills are all important. Competence remains a key issue at all levels of practice. For ophthalmic nurses striving towards advanced practice, this will mean being involved in strategic planning for eye services both locally and nationally, taking the lead in practice development, being autonomous practitioners, and instigating evidence-based changes in practice (RCN 2012).

Health education

The need to promote ocular health has been emphasised in this book as an important competence to demonstrate when managing the care of older people with age-related ocular diseases (RCN 2012). In the future, health and social care professionals will need to continue to contribute to the dissemination of ocular public health information, promote the UK Vision Strategy (2013–2018) and generally educate the public by raising awareness of government strategies.

With specific reference to cataract, AMD, glaucoma and diabetic retinopathy, providing information and advice about the significance of the relationship between lifestyle and eye disease is an important part of the health and social care professional's role as a health educator. Dietary intake, alcohol consumption, exercise levels and smoking have all been advanced as significant risk factors in the development of eye disease. Furthermore, the provision and uptake of eye care and screening services have also been stressed as aids to the early detection of abnormalities and provision of appropriate treatment.

Psychosocial role

The psychosocial role is also very important, since the onset of depression in the visually impaired older person, as well as family carers, has social and economic implications. Counselling skills are needed to help older people and their families deal with the shock of visual loss and to provide a basis for subsequent patient empowerment (Watkinson 2011).

Exploring and understanding the reasons for depression associated with sight loss is critical in trying to facilitate this process. Self-sufficiency and self-esteem are diminished as a person mourns the loss of their ability to see (Watkinson 2011). In this situation, the use of psychosocial theory can be invaluable to the caring practitioner. The use of social cognitive models can facilitate the exploration of the older person's health beliefs and attitudes and help to explain how the impact of sight loss has caused the behavioural changes leading to depression. More importantly, such models will also provide strategies for starting to make positive behavioural changes for the future (Watkinson 2011).

Conclusion

In summary, managing the care of older people with visual impairment will pose challenges for the future due to the UK's changing demography. The inevitable increased incidence of ocular disease, such as cataract, AMD, COAG, and diabetic retinopathy, will necessitate serious consideration of the future financial burden of visual impairment in the UK. We therefore need to invest in identifying sight problems at an early stage and initiating treatment where possible. This will help reduce future demand for more complex and costly support from the health and social care system and will improve quality of life for older people with visual problems.

Overall, ophthalmic nurses and all relevant health and social care professionals will need to demonstrate professional behaviour, intrinsic motivation and commitment to ongoing participation in professional education to increase their professional knowledge base and advance their practice. Undeniably, technological advances, specialist nurses and the competent delivery of technical skills are all pivotal to achieving successful delivery of care to older patients with visual impairment. But these advances must not be achieved at the expense of a compassionate, caring relationship between practitioner and patient.

Political awareness and strong leadership skills are needed to argue for more resources for the care and management of older people with visual impairment. Consequently, the importance of current knowledge of public health issues, government healthcare policies, legal and ethical issues, significant professional developments and evidence-based practice cannot be underestimated. The research role and the need to continue to expand the scientific evidence base related to caring practice should also be prioritised.

Future perspective

The implications of continued financial constraint over the next decade may mean that the UK government is unable to meet the key NHS priorities for the care of older people with visual impairment. Such pressures have already resulted in a worrying decline in some standards of care. Money is now being saved by employing healthcare assistants and support workers, rather than more highly qualified staff, within the NHS. This in turn has led to an urgent need to provide a training programme that will equip such practitioners with the knowledge and skills required to provide basic care and services. This proposed training is currently being considered, and it is to be hoped that positive decisions will emerge that will ensure the future provision of good-quality care for older people with visual impairment.

References

Alzheimer's Society (2013). 'Number of people with dementia in minority ethnic groups could rise seven fold by 2051 and yet awareness and support is lacking.' (News article) http://www.alzheimers.org.uk/site/scripts/news_article. php?newsID=1659 (last accessed: 20 January 2014).

Department of Health (2009). *Living Well with Dementia: A National Dementia Strategy.* London: DH.

Department of Health (2012). *Compassion in Practice. Nursing Midwifery and Care Staff. Our Vision and Strategy.* London: NHS Commissioning Board.

Department of Health (2013). *Independent Inquiry into care provided by Mid Staffordshire NHS Foundation Trust: January 2005–March 2009.* The Mid Staffordshire NHS Foundation Trust Public Inquiry: The Francis Report. London: DH.

Diabetes UK (2012). DIABETES IN THE UK 2012: Key statistics on diabetes. www.diabetes.org.uk/Documents/ Reports/Diabetes-in-the-UK-2012.pdf (Last accessed: 28 April 2014).

Kanski, J. & Bowling, B. (2011). *Clinical Ophthalmology: A Systematic Approach.* 7th edn. London: Elsevier.

National Health and Social Care Information Centre (2011a). Hospital prescribing: England 2010. NHSIC. Available at www.hscic.gov.uk (Search term: 'hospital prescribing; England 2010, Last accessed: 28 April 2014).

National Health and Social Care Information Centre (2011b). 'Hospital Episode Statistics: Inpatient headline summary, 2010/11 NHSIC' in *Eye Health data summary 2012. A review of published data in England.* www.orthoptics.org.uk/ Resources/Documents/Eye%20health%20data%20summary%202012%20-%20England.pdf (Last accessed: 28 April 2014).

National Health and Social Care Information Centre (2011c). *Prescription Costs Analysis Information Centre: England, 2010.* NHSIC. www.ic.nhs.uk/statistics-and-data-collections (Last accessed: 13 July 2013).

National Institute of Clinical Excellence (2009). *Glaucoma: diagnosis and management of chronic open-angle glaucoma and ocular hypertension.* NICE Clinical Guideline 85. London: NICE.

National Screening Committee (2012). *English National Screening Programme for Diabetic Retinopathy: Annual Report, 2010/11.* UK National Screening Committee. www.diabeticeye.screening.nhs.uk (Last accessed: 13 July 2013).

Nursing and Midwifery Council (2009). *Guidance: for care of older people.* London: NMC.

Polack, S. (2008). Restoring sight: how cataract surgery improves the lives of older adults. *Community Eye Health.* **21** (66), 24–25.

Riordan-Eva, P. & Whitcher, J. (2008). *Vaughan and Asbury's General Ophthalmology.* 17th edn. New York, NY, USA: Lange Medical Books/McGraw-Hill.

Royal College of Nursing (2012). *Ophthalmic nursing: an integrated career and competence framework.* London: RCN.

Royal National Institute of Blind People (2009). *Low vision service outcomes: a systematic review.* Low Vision Service Model Evaluation (LOVSME) Project. London: RNIB.

Royal National Institute of Blind People (2013a). *UK Vision Strategy 2013–2018 – Vision2020 UK.* www.vision2020uk.org. uk/ukvisionstrategy/core/core_picker/download.asp?id=539&filetitle=UK+Vision (Last accessed: 27 April 2014).

Royal National Institute of Blind People (2013b) Sight loss UK 2013. The latest evidence. www.rnib.org.uk/sites/default/ files/ Sight_loss_UK_2013_pdf (Last accessed: 27 April 2014).

UK National Statistics Publication Hub (2014). 'Older People'. Available at www.statistics.gov.uk (Search term 'older people'. Last accessed: 27 April 2014).

Watkinson, S. (2009). Management of visual impairment in older people: what can the nurse do? *Ageing Health.* **5** (6), 821–32.

Watkinson, S. (2011). Managing depression in older people with visual impairment. *Nursing Older People.* **23** (8), 23–28.

World Health Organisation (2013). 'About Diabetes'. www.who.int/diabetes/action_online/basics/en/index3.html (Last accessed: 3 July 2013).

Index